DRE...
—— AND THE ——
INNER SELF

Ray Douglas

BLANDFORD

A BLANDFORD BOOK

First published in the UK 1999
by Blandford
A Cassell imprint

Cassell plc
Wellington House
125 Strand
London WC2R 0BB

www.cassell.co.uk

Distributed in the United States by Sterling Publishing Co., Inc.,
387 Park Avenue South, New York, NY 10016-8810

A Cataloguing-in-Publication Data entry for this title is available and may be
obtained from the British Library

ISBN 0-7137-2776-4

Designed by Chris Bell
Printed in Great Britain by MPG Books Ltd., Bodmin, Cornwall

CONTENTS

THE DREAMING SELF

DREAMS IN THEIR DEVELOPMENT HAVE BREATH,
AND TEARS, AND TORTURES, AND THE TOUCH OF JOY;
THEY LEAVE A WEIGHT UPON OUR WAKING THOUGHTS,
THEY TAKE A WEIGHT FROM OFF OUR WAKING TOILS.
THEY DO DIVIDE OUR BEING; THEY BECOME
A PORTION OF OURSELVES AS OF OUR TIME,
AND LOOK LIKE HERALDS OF ETERNITY.

George Gordon, Lord Byron

A DREAM sometimes seems like an onion with many layers: we can't sample the onion simply by looking at its outer skin. In order to understand the language, the symbolism, the imagery of a dream, we need first to look more deeply until we find its hidden nature; and to understand the hidden nature of dreams, we need to learn something about the nature of the dreaming self.

The whole self is also rather like an onion: it includes more than the outer skin of appearance, the body, thoughts, emotions and sensations; the self is more than the ego, more than personality, more even than individuality; it is more, too, than the simple sum of all these parts. The self includes the unconscious as well as the conscious mind; the male sex as well as the female; transmitting channel as well as receptive vessel.

We can quite accurately think of the whole self as a circle – or, more correctly, as a globe or a sphere. Forget, for a moment, the human form of flesh, bones and blood; we have to consider the self as an independent entity without a material body to contain it. Your dreams are not limited to the confines of your body and of your brain. While a person is dreaming, their own personal sphere is potentially that much more complete, for it is on the way to wholeness. 'Wholeness' is

5

something that we, as fallible creatures, don't really understand. But we know instinctively, at a very deep level, that wholeness is the goal – the direction in which we should all be heading.

You can well imagine that something whole and alive, yet lacking in materiality, will take the form of a sphere. Even material things take this perfect shape, when circumstances allow, rather like a bubble, or the sun, or a planet revolving around it in space. It is the path of least resistance; any flexible entity without outside influences yet with its own centre of gravity is likely to adopt this spherical form. It is, per-haps, as fundamental and abstract a state of being as one can imagine. But even this abstract state of selfhood as a non-material sphere can be reflected in dreams, as this example shows:

> ℂ I seemed to be floating in space, and all around were orbs like bright bubbles, glowing with different colours which seemed to move and flow like water or oil, like rainbows shimmering, both inside and out. It was all very beautiful and peaceful. Then I became aware of a 'black hole', a frightening, dark presence which threatened to swal-low up anything in its path. There was no way I could escape, so I just sat or floated there in space. Then the 'black hole' passed over me and disappeared; I still felt perfectly calm and peaceful, because it could not harm me at all.

There is really nothing further to be analysed, or interpreted, in a dream of this nature. The feeling of weightlessness, of floating, of peace and beauty, and a complete lack of materiality to anchor the self to earth, is fundamental to life. In waking life we think, and we feel, and these functions conceal our unconscious minds and our inner feelings. Our inner feelings do not, *as a rule*, come to our awareness, but it is their function to create or select the images which are remembered as dreams. These inner feelings that dream, not being encumbered by the physical body, can travel where they will, and even float freely in space. They are not attached to materiality. In our dreams we can fly, and often do.

The 'black hole' in the dream example above, certainly, may have been suggested to the dreamer's conscious mind by something that was in itself material – something disturbing that may have been experi-enced or read about. Quite possibly it was the horrific prospect of an actual 'black hole' in space, said to be able to swallow up whole galax-ies – but in this dream its dark image was conjured up and used to demonstrate the fact that materiality has no effect on the transcendental self. And the self is certainly greater than the merely psychological contents of the personality, which may sometimes seem in our imagination to be on the point of devouring it. Often it seems the more 'advanced' a dream is, the more 'basic' will its nature be, for development of the self involves shedding a great deal of unnecessary psychological clutter.

A HOLISTIC MANDALA

The first diagram resembles a wheel within a wheel, or a globe within a globe. This kind of diagram is a mandala – a Sanskrit word meaning 'magic circle' – representing the self. Inside this mandala is the familiar, everyday 'self', small-scale and personal, the wide-awake experience of awareness – as well as the unconscious, sleeping part of this personal self: the inner feelings, which belong to what Jung called the 'personal unconscious'. The larger, encompassing wheel must still be thought of as part of the 'self' – this time the greater self, including mysterious areas that often do not seem to be part of ourselves at all:

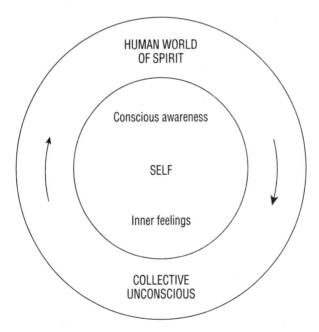

A diagram of the self as an abstract idea: the personal within the greater impersonal. Matters which are normally unconscious can come to our awareness in dreams.

7

the 'collective unconscious' (Jung's term again), and the human world of spirit, which is directly linked to universal spirit.

These greater contents or principles are shared equally by the whole of humankind, so taken together they can be called the 'impersonal self'. Neither the collective unconscious nor the human world of spirit is fixed or restricted, or isolated from the rest of creation. There is a constant flow or interchange beyond our normal experience, between the ordinary self of conscious awareness with its thoughts and feelings, and the inner feelings of the personal unconscious; and there is also a link between the greater self, the world of the collective unconscious, and the world of human spirit.

The first of these connections, or channels of communication, gives rise to what we might call everyday dreams, associated with our normal lives and the people with whom we come into daily contact, and occasionally also to deeper dreams informing us of our own hidden contents, which may have been influencing our thoughts and behaviour from within. Under certain circumstances, the flow of information from the greater impersonal world of the unconscious can also come to the awareness of the ordinary self, and when this happens our dreams occupy a different dimension, take on a new urgency, and carry a more vivid and insistent message.

Let us take a closer look at the 'ordinary self' – at ourselves – and see how this constant interchange of contents, this fluid movement of information, actually works. Again, we must picture the self as it might be, if there were no such thing as a physical body, no material influences, and no gravitational pull to influence it. We can realistically believe now that people were created 'in God's image', for a universal creator would have to encompass his entire universe and, being utterly whole and non-material, could only be envisaged as a sphere, or globe, containing all globes and all movements.

But, of course, very few people are really whole, either spiritually or psychologically. The first step towards progress is to understand our limitations. Most of us would admit that we are flawed, in one way or another, at least to the extent that we are *not* aware of everything; not open to everything. We are not even directly aware of our own contents, never mind our true place in the universe. Perhaps this is why we need dreams, to help us along. It has been said that truly whole people have no further need for dreams, for they are already aware of all these things, and all the possibilities open to them. But for all of *us*, as we are being realistic, dreams are the next best thing; if we let them, they will carry us in the right direction.

THE PERSONAL SHADOW

The second mandala diagram gives an idea of how the process works at the personal dream level. The circle here represents the sphere of the personal self. The horizontal line – the horizon – represents the division between day, or all that is known to the conscious mind, above, and night, or all that is unknown and mysterious, below. Remember the cyclic process that works continuously beneath the level of awareness, carrying impulses and influences from one part of the sphere to another. In the waking, daylight zone, the normal everyday feelings are surrounded, in effect, by a shell representing the thinking mind. In sleep, this shell disappears, or softens.

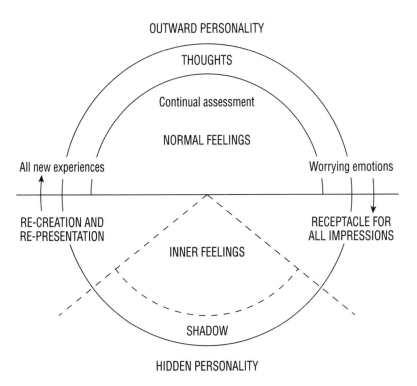

A diagram of the dreaming self. Impressions gathered during the day sink into the unconscious mind, where worries and problems are worked upon, analysed and reassembled by the inner feelings, to re-emerge in the form of dreams and waking inspirations.

In the darkest part of the hidden side of the personality, the personal shadow collects beneath the inner feelings, as though pulled down and gathered there by the gravity of materiality. This is the part of personality that people tend to disown, and fail to recognize as their own if it should try to come to awareness. It contains everything pertaining to ourselves that we might think of as undesirable, or unlovable, or downright evil. It represent the night-time Mr Hyde as the *alter ego* of the day-time Dr Jekyll.

In Chinese philosophy, these two halves of the personal globe are called *yin* and *yang*; the masculine and positive element of *yang* in the light, the feminine and negative element of *yin* in the darkness. During the course of the day our thoughts and feelings, as the objective *yang*, are constantly assessing everything that comes to their notice. Things they dislike, or find they cannot readily cope with because they are too negative or subjective, tend to be disowned and pushed away. But these unwanted contents do not simply disappear; they sink down into the inner feelings – and may even add to the burden of the personal shadow, lurking in the depths of the negative *yin*.

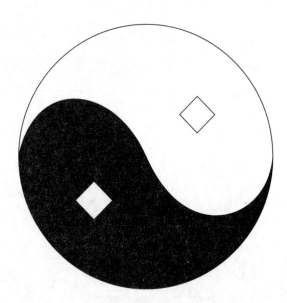

A diagram of the universal self in Chinese philosophy. The bright awareness of the positive yang *rides above the dark unconsciousness of the negative* yin.

10

Whether they are acceptable to the conscious mind or not, all the experiences and impressions of each day, or their memories, eventually filter down through the evening horizon, via the male channel of the *yang*, into the female receptacle of the *yin*. There everything is collected, collated, processed and stored within the inner feelings. Much of this material is reassembled or re-created, perhaps with a new slant. It may be given a completely unsuspected significance, a new shade of meaning, or a conclusion that had been overlooked by the conscious mind. These are the new understandings, the inspirations, that are presented or re-presented to the waking mind in a more readily assimilable form, They may come to the awareness during waking hours as a vision or sudden inspiration; but more commonly they are received as dreams.

We may well have learnt at school that the seventeenth-century mathematician and philosopher Descartes actually dreamed the basic principles of analytical geometry, and on waking put his inspiration into practice; and that the nineteenth-century writer Robert Louis Stevenson said that he used to dream the plots of his novels. *The Strange Case of Dr Jekyll and Mr Hyde*, which I have already mentioned as an example of the personal shadow taking a tangible form, was the outcome of one of these dreams. Cases such as these of practical, constructive dreams are only well known because they refer to famous people, who happened to notice and were prepared to admit the important part which dreams had played in their lives; but this type of inspiration, this dream-education, is by no means limited to outstanding or exceptionally gifted people. It happens to almost all of us most of the time, whether we are aware of it or not.

The essence and aim of the Chinese system of working with *yin* and *yang* is to achieve the *Tao*, the path to wholeness, through an even balance of these two opposite but complementary principles. You will see that when an even balance, an equal assimilation of the two, has been achieved, the need for continual cycling (or dreaming) will no longer be there. Even the shadow will have become accepted and re-assimilated; perfect 'individuation' will have taken place, and the individual will indeed be a whole, untroubled human being, without psychological problems.

Once some sort of start has been made along the path to wholeness, and personal assimilation of the *yin* along with the *yang* has begun, dreams can change their nature. They may warn of the daily need to deal with matters positively as they reach the conscious mind, rather than to pursue the old negative, if unconscious, habit of pushing them away into the dark. You will recall this matter when you reach the latter part of the book. The following is a typical dream warning against misuse of the 'receptacle for all impressions':

⊄ In my dream there was a hole in the garden, about 12 feet deep and 6 feet across, into which we had always been accustomed to throw our rubbish in the past. I went outside with a screwed up piece of old, dirty clothing in my hand, and threw it into the pit. There were two men standing by the side of the pit, and they shouted at me crossly: 'We've just cleared this pit out, and you are not to throw any more rubbish into it!' They said I must go down into the pit and clean it out myself. I said I couldn't do that, and felt very alarmed because they were belligerent, and if I went down into the pit, I did not see how I could climb out again. I woke up feeling frightened.

DON'T BLOCK YOURSELF OUT

Whether you follow any particular religion or not, you will tend to have one of two distinct 'attitudes' towards higher things – towards impersonal spiritual powers. Either you will metaphorically bow your head to what may be, get on with everyday life and submit your final destiny into those unknown higher hands – or you will try to influence or even control your own spiritual destiny. You may even follow some system involving work on the self, using meditation or yogic concentration designed to keep out 'unwanted influences'. But influences can be good as well as bad, and you cannot tell which is which until you actually feel them; the healthy cycle of dreams depends on the acceptance and free interchange of influences within the self.

Serious meditation may tend to close off access to the personal unconscious. When this happens, awareness of your own dark contents is no longer possible, so you may come to believe they are no longer there. You may even begin to create your own predictably agreeable, self-approving dreams, the products of your own desire, and this really would be a step backwards on the path of life. You will see why this has to be so when you study the concept of the world dream (see Chapter 3). You need to allow your dreams free rein, because they are able to transcend your own desires, and your own intentions.

Studied intentions and determination are always necessary for material achievement, and this is the direction in which they should be aimed. But this natural cycle of dreams is working to lead the self in the opposite direction, towards the possibility of submissive psychic wholeness rather than added material strength. Conscious efforts to alter the quality of consciousness, or any movement that is 'power orientated', inevitably set up a counter-flow. If asked, then, I should advise against trying to 'float untroubled like a lotus flower'. Remain open to your own contents at all times, for they are part of the whole you.

THE DREAMING PROCESS

Many people forget their dreams so thoroughly they deny ever dreaming at all; but this, of course, is not the same as actually having no dreams. If you genuinely have no dreams, you are unlikely to be reading this book. But if, like many others, you merely find it difficult or impossible to remember your dreams, you have been missing out on a chance to experience an amazingly direct method of learning and understanding things that are normally unknown to our conscious minds. I hope that through reading this book, you will find that remembering and understanding your dreams soon comes naturally to you.

When you can remember and understand your *personal* dreams, those resulting from the reassembled, re-created and re-presented impressions of normal awareness – a second bite of the cherry which would otherwise not be available to you – then you will begin to experience *impersonal* dreams, even dream messages from the human world of spirit. These are truly instructive, meaningful experiences: spiritual truths coming to awareness, things you ought to know but could not otherwise discover; experiences that will guarantee you are never quite the same person again.

The fourth mandala diagram (overleaf) makes it plain that the nature of dreams tends to vary according to the hour of dreaming, or, equally, to your own mental state when you experience the dream. The mandala can be seen as a clock, divided into day and night. You do not really, of course, go to sleep at sunset and wake up on the dot at sunrise, but do not let this obvious fact disguise the truth of the mandala itself. After waking in the morning, by the broad light of noon you are normally at your most wide awake. Evening sees you wearied of the day's toing and froing – whether you actually lead a hectically busy life or not; it doesn't matter.

Everything that the conscious mind has assimilated, enjoyed, or dwelled upon, or pretended not to notice, or actively ignored, or rejected and disowned, all these impressions are submitted by the now

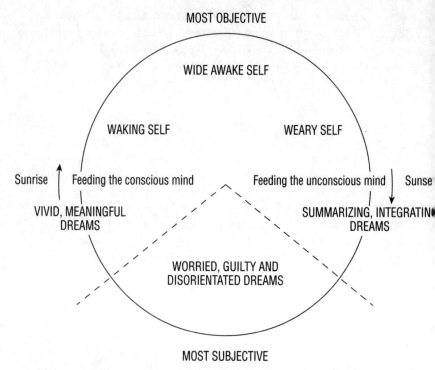

MOST OBJECTIVE

WIDE AWAKE SELF

WAKING SELF   WEARY SELF

Sunrise ↑ Feeding the conscious mind   Feeding the unconscious mind ↓ Sunse

VIVID, MEANINGFUL
DREAMS
     SUMMARIZING, INTEGRATIN
DREAMS

WORRIED, GUILTY AND
DISORIENTATED DREAMS

MOST SUBJECTIVE

All the impressions of the day sink into subconsciousness in a disorganized jumble, gradually becoming co-ordinated by the unconscious mind during sleep. Our dreams tend to reflect this continuing process at work.

weary mind into the realms of the unconscious. There, they become food for the personal unconscious, and this part of the mind functioning beneath the horizon of awareness continues to work through the night, through your sleeping hours, summarizing, comparing, identifying similarities and categorizing them, integrating all your thoughts, feelings and sensations into a fresh viewpoint, a new understanding.

Dozing dreams – those that appear of an instant as soon as you close your eyes and nod off in your chair – are still in a dissembled state, still in the process of integration, and they will seldom make sense when you snap our of your doze and recall them. They will probably bear a semblance of waking thoughts and observations but, jumbled, they will never quite make sense. They are infant dreams in the making. This is a typically 'trivial', evening dream:

⦿ There was a row of circular white seats arranged along what seemed to be the ridge of a hill; it might have been overlooking a waterfall. They seemed to be slowly sliding down the rocks at different speeds. I was sitting on one of them, and it was moving faster than the others. It was all very obscure.

On waking, the dreamer was not sure whether the circular objects *were* in fact seats after all – they might have been some sticky labels that she had been using during the day. And she was not sure whether anybody else was actually sitting on them or not. So, whatever they were, and whatever they represented, this was not really meant even to *be* a dream; it was merely a brief glimpse of the procession of events, memories and impressions, as they passed down into the subconscious – the personal unconscious mind. By itself, the dream picture was meaningless to the conscious mind, however interpreted.

Dreams develop and grow as time passes. In the middle of the night – or in the middle, at least, of the sleeping state – remembered dreams tend to be more complicated, indeed more meaningful, but seldom either conclusive or pleasant. By this stage of the process the varied impressions which they consist of will have been identified and resolved into their true nature, their most appropriate form as products of the weary self: maybe things you would rather not face; worries that you have pushed to the back of your mind. Dreams are working towards wholeness, and these matters need to be dealt with. Here they are all in vivid pictorial form: the worries, the fears, the guilt, all clearly visible. But at this time they represent problems that have *not* yet been solved, worries that have not yet been put into a positive light; they are still in the process of resolution and re-creation.

⦿ I was in a small wood with bluebells and primroses growing among the bushes. I felt I was being followed and looked round in alarm, and saw several mentally disabled men coming after me and obviously trying to catch me. The wood now seemed full of thorns and brambles, but I found that I could walk on or run along the tops of these prickly bushes to escape. My husband woke me at this point, as I had been throwing myself about in the bed.

This dream is a typical expression of an unresolved problem, a series of worries or unhelpful attitudes. I would not attempt to analyse it: it seems the dreamer was awakened too soon, otherwise the dream itself would probably not have been remembered. If allowed to continue or recur through the rest of the night, a solution to whatever was troubling the conscious mind of the dreamer might well have emerged, towards dawn. Just before dawn, you will find, is the time for vivid, really meaningful dreams to emerge in their completed form. Timed to coincide with waking, they are *intended* to be remembered. Solution and re-creation, if it is to take place at all with the available material, will by then be complete.

Fear of the unknown, or possibly, as in the last example, fear of mental disorder, or perhaps fear of strangers, or foreigners – this type of problem is likely to be focused upon and resolved by way of a dawn dream. To illustrate this, an example of a dream denouncing the folly of racial prejudice is given here. It should be explained that this dream happened during the era of Mao Tse-tung's cultural revolution when, at one time, to most people's bafflement, Chinese nationals in their European embassies sometimes seemed determined to provoke aggressive confrontation with uninvolved and normally completely uninterested passers-by.

> I dreamed of a shadowy oriental figure, and felt very threatened by him. I seized a long pole with a basket tied to the end – the sort of thing that occasionally features in Chinese paintings of peasant life – and began to belabour the shadowy figure about the head with it. Suddenly, I saw that he was not Chinese, nor was he at all threatening; he was an elderly Indonesian gentleman (whom I knew in real life), for whom I had the greatest respect. He was laughing at my mistake as he warded off my blows, and I felt dreadfully ashamed of my unreasonable behaviour. I felt that I would never again allow myself to misunderstand or pre-judge people on the basis of racial differences. This was a dawn dream.

This dream falls into the category: 'fear of an unknown assailant', a device often used by the dreaming self. In this case, it is brought to a successful and very worthwhile conclusion: a conclusion that builds character out of chaos, and produces brotherly love where only fear and suspicion existed before. Further interpretation is not required; this is the very best sort of personal dream.

16

ANALYSE YOUR OWN DREAMS

HERE AM I, FINGERING MY WORKERS TO THE BONE,
AND ALL YOU DO IS DREAM!

Pantomime, *Jack and the Beanstalk*

A DREAM is a story – a pantomime, even. Remember the story of your dream. Think around it carefully; go through the whole sequence in your mind; write it down with every detail you can remember. Draw it if you like – you don't have to be an artist. It will help if you list the details separately, in the correct order. Look first at the general story; then look between the details – read between the lines. Every story has a theme, or more than one theme, to carry it along. Try to recall the theme and the emotions which carried the details along in your dream.

Your feelings during and immediately after the dream are important pointers. You might remember feeling happy as you experienced one dream detail, sad when you experienced another. You may have felt anxious, annoyed, relieved, worried, pleased, angry, puzzled, amused – all these feelings are significant if you want to reveal the true meaning of your dream.

PERSONAL DREAMS; PERSONAL IMAGES

On the surface, a complicated dream might have more than one meaning, or sets of meanings. Like a fairytale, there is often a deeper story hidden within the more obvious one. The number of meanings a dream may have is indeterminate. Dreams are symbol-based, and symbols can represent more than one thing at once. Their meaning depends on what they mean to *you*. The deepest meaning is probably the one that has the greatest significance for you.

A personal dream reflects the circumstances which have given rise to it, the things that have happened to you, and your reactions to them. If your dream is personal, its contents will be personal too, and for your eyes and ears alone. Non-personal dreams have far greater, wider meanings – meanings that may have arisen from a collective source. Collective dreams will be filled with more than your own personal contents, and when you experience this type of dream, you will probably be left in no doubt about the meaning. If they too are obscure, some of the other chapters in this book will help you to understand them. But at least ninety-nine out of every hundred dreams you experience will relate to you; your own experiences; your own reactions; and, often enough, your own deeply considered advice to yourself.

Our minds are miraculously complicated and finely balanced, and capable of great things. But our everyday thoughts are not usually the product of the *highest* part of our minds. We all have similar tendencies: we justify our thoughts, our actions, our attitudes, our foibles. If we could only use the higher parts of our mind all the time, our reactions and feelings would probably be quite different. It is the higher, or deeper, part of our own self that can let itself be known during the process of remembering dreams.

No matter how complicated the details, the message a dream carries can be quite straightforward, merely expressing some worry that you have put to the back of your mind. Write down the dream story in simple, straightforward terms:

€ In the dream I was upstairs with my brother. I looked out of a window and saw two young men acting suspiciously in the garden. One was wearing a mask. My brother said, 'Oh well, they're going to break in, I expect,' and he didn't seem at all worried. In fact, he then went to bed. I was agitated for what seemed some time through the night. I don't know whose house it was, but I think our mother was in there somewhere. Then I heard a break-in happening downstairs. I could also hear the sound of water running and splashing. I tried to telephone the police, but the operator said: 'Sorry, there is a hold-up. You cannot contact the police for about forty minutes.' I decided to confront the intruders, and wondered what weapon I could use, but could find nothing suitable. Then I was downstairs, feeling threatened, and made to sit on the floor against a wall. One of the intruders was carrying a saw-like tool. I was afraid they might torture us. A dog looked in through the door briefly, and then went away again. I remember thinking, 'I don't care what they do to me, but I couldn't stand it if they tortured the dog!' (In fact we do not have a dog, and neither does my mother.)

It is a good idea to make out a personal questionnaire. List all the elements of the dream in sequence and, by following your own association of ideas, your own train of thought, write down in turn everything these details remind you of. Do the same with the themes, if they are at all identifiable. Again, write down anything these secondary elements and themes remind you of, as though following a new storyline for each item, until you run out of ideas. When this happens, return to the general picture of your dream and think again. Let your mind spin little incidental stories if you like, but concentrate on the memories that the dream has conjured up. If you feel that a particular train of thought is becoming too unpleasant to continue, it is best to persevere anyway – you could be approaching something significant that your 'everyday' mind is trying to hide. Even if it shows you up in a bad light, no one else will know! It is your own private dream, after all, and intended for you alone. It will help if you can turn your thoughts and memories into an organized diagram, too, showing each connection in turn until you reach a conclusion (see overleaf).

Whose house?   Not mine; I live in a bungalow. I'm sure it was mother's house, though there seemed to be no familiar details. I had been on the phone to her that day, and I had a feeling that she was there, in the dream.
Two men?   They were skulking about and obviously up to no good.
One with a mask?   He obviously didn't want to be recognized. It could have been someone known to us, or more probably, someone already known to mother.
Brother went to bed?   He seemed very complacent, but that's how he is in real life! No sense of danger or urgency. It made me feel it was my own personal responsibility, but I also felt quite helpless.
Sound of water?   Mother recently had trouble with the main cistern, and had to call a neighbour to help. I could have been remembering that. The incident showed that when things go wrong she has to rely on outsiders.
Break-in?   In the dream I knew this was happening downstairs. I felt vulnerable but responsible, with no one else available to help.
Tried to phone police?   It reminds me of the only time I ever tried to call the police for a real emergency, and the emergency services let me down badly on that occasion. They probably took about forty minutes to arrive.

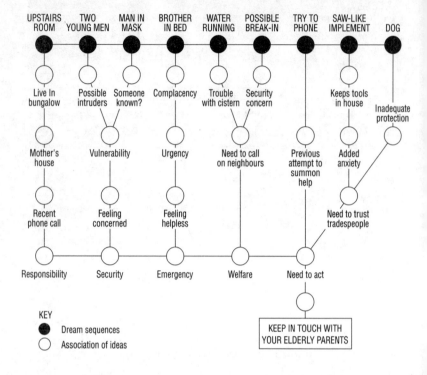

Saw-like tool? Mother often has various tradespeople doing work in the house or the garden. She keeps various tools in the house, that used to belong to father, so I suppose there is a security risk here.

Dog? I can't make any real sense out of this, except to stress that there is no 'guard-dog' protection, and no deterrent for intending intruders.

Themes: Lack of security; complacency; suspicion; vulnerability; helplessness.

Conclusion: As we live a hundred miles apart, it is difficult to see what I can do, other than keep in touch regularly. Mother has another son who lives much nearer, and he ought to call in more regularly.

Having completed your questionnaire and the diagram, look at some of the points again from a non-personal angle. There might be another, more cryptic meaning. Try not to rationalize your dream experiences and answers too much; follow them through as if you were listening to a story about someone else. This way you won't spare the feelings of the dream characters, and you are less likely to spare your own feelings. Analyse your own answers. Recall your own relationships with the other dream characters – especially any unpleasant memories and recent experiences. Only you can remember your own feelings during and after the dream: decide how they fit into the story.

Who is that masked intruder again; could it be you, the dreamer, intruding in some other sense? And how about that dog. Could this again be a projection of your own attitude? Your dreams may be revealing the true *you* without your familiar mask or disguise – or they may be portraying you as others are sometimes liable to see you, and you may not recognize yourself.

Breaking the rules

If you felt guilty at any stage in your dream, this may be because you have been breaking the rules in real life – your *own* rules of morality and fair play. This sort of rule-breaking, denying your conscience, is often at the root of disturbing dreams. The moral is, we all need to be true to our own sense of morality. There is a certain amount of guilt at the back of the dream in the next example:

> € I was walking through a large empty building, and wanted to go downstairs to go home. Somebody had left a filing cabinet in the way and that made me feel very cross. I pushed it as I walked past, but it wouldn't move and I nearly fell down a lift shaft. There was no lift, just an open shaft, but this did not seem surprising to me in the dream. I wanted to go down the shaft, but decided not to. I looked through a window and saw my boyfriend and my boss, laughing and joking together. Then I was at home with my little sister, who was being difficult. She kicked me on the shin, and said, 'I'll tell mummy!' A door opened then, and the sound of loud music came through. I opened a window to 'let the sound out', and saw two pennies on the window-sill.

Empty building? I think it was supposed to be the building where I work. It felt empty and cheerless, which is how I feel about work just now.
Filing cabinet? This definitely makes me think of work. There are stacks of filing cabinets there. I tried to move this one and it wouldn't move. There are a lot of things I'd like to change at work, and can't!
Somebody had left it in the way? Things have not been going well at work. The people there have been awkward. All right, I suppose I have been awkward as well. But nothing seems to go right, and I suppose I was feeling

21

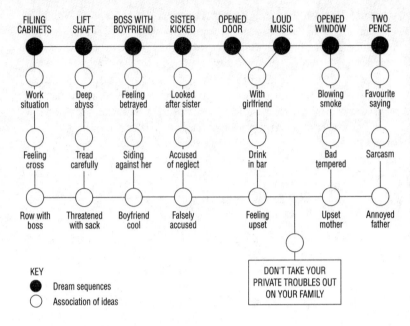

FILING CABINETS	LIFT SHAFT	BOSS WITH BOYFRIEND	SISTER KICKED	OPENED DOOR	LOUD MUSIC	OPENED WINDOW	TWO PENCE
Work situation	Deep abyss	Feeling betrayed	Looked after sister	With girlfriend		Blowing smoke	Favourite saying
Feeling cross	Tread carefully	Siding against her	Accused of neglect	Drink in bar		Bad tempered	Sarcasm
Row with boss	Threatened with sack	Boyfriend cool	Falsely accused	Feeling upset		Upset mother	Annoyed father

KEY
● Dream sequences
○ Association of ideas

DON'T TAKE YOUR PRIVATE TROUBLES OUT ON YOUR FAMILY

cross about it. I recently had a row with the boss, and I was thinking about looking for another job anyway.

Open lift shaft? There was a danger of falling in and getting hurt. It meant I had to tread carefully. After my row with the boss I was in danger of getting the sack, and perhaps that is what it referred to. It is still a possibility, and I would certainly not like that. If I leave the job I would rather go voluntarily.

Boss and boyfriend together? My boyfriend is a salesman connected with the same firm. When I told him about my tiff with the boss he seemed to think it was my fault. I felt a bit let down. As I see it he was siding with the enemy.

Kicked by little sister? I don't know why she should be spiteful. I've done nothing to her. But I was looking after her the other day, and had to stay in when I would rather be going out. There was a bit of a misunderstanding, so when mother came home she thought I'd been neglectful, but I hadn't. My little sister could have spoken up for me, but she didn't – of course!

Open door? Loud music? I think this followed on from the last incident. The loud music was probably when I went out with a girlfriend and we had a few drinks, and I came back late. It was a reaction. I was still feeling fed up, and of course my parents didn't care for that at all.

Opened window? When I got home my mother made a remark about me smoking and blowing smoke, so I opened a window rather sarcastically. I think this is what it must refer to.

Two pennies? I can't think why coins should have significance. But later on I remembered that father has a favourite saying: 'I don't give tuppence for . . .' whatever it is he's complaining about. I suppose he wasn't really complaining, but he was probably feeling annoyed. I suppose my behaviour towards them hasn't been all that good.

Themes: Feeling at odds with everyone else. Bad temper.

Conclusion: It does look as if my private problems have been affecting my relationship with my parents and friends. I accept that the dream could be dropping me a hint.

Parts of yourself

Everything you do, and particularly everything about your relationships that you dislike, or cannot understand, or that your emotions cannot easily cope with, finds its way down into your subconscious. You may have forgotten about something, but it has not really been forgotten. It is liable to emerge into awareness again, and the way in which it does this depends upon your own attitude. Are you basically positive or negative? Do you see yourself as a problem person, or as a growing and developing one – a potentially whole person?

Frightening dreams usually point to a problem which is inside us. If we heed dreams like this and try to understand them, they may supply us with the motivation we need if we are to face up to and deal with these hidden problems. When you begin to observe and record your own dreams, you will probably meet an opposing influence of some sort, symbolized as a villain, a demon, a devil, a witch, a nameless frightener. This dark presence is probably a part of yourself, which should be released and not contained. Let it come out if it will.

> In my dream I was waiting for my boyfriend John to arrive, because I wanted him to meet a special person – a lady who was staying with me, a very sweet person. When John arrived I rushed to open the door, but in my haste I caused the lady to fall downstairs. I shouted at John to go away while I rushed downstairs to help the lady, but John came in. I didn't want him to see what was going on, so I tried to stop him going downstairs. By then the lady had disappeared, but there was something dark and unpleasant down there, and it seemed important to me that John should not see it. He was bringing me some

23

flowers, and I was carrying a vase in my hand, but I wouldn't let him put the flowers in it. He looked down the stairs and said: 'What's that down there?' I said, 'It's only the boiler!' Then to stop him going down the stairs I grabbed the flowers and started to hit him with them, shouting, 'Get out!' I woke up then feeling angry and sorry at the same time.

John's arrival? I felt glad, not because I wanted to see John, exactly, but because I wanted him to meet my lady friend. I thought he would find her attractive and interesting.

The lady fell downstairs? It was my fault. She was so sweet and harmless, and I knocked her flying when all I wanted to do was introduce her to John.

Why did I like the lady so much? I don't know. She just seemed someone I could admire, and I felt very attached to her. She had a sweet face. I remember now that she had a small mole on her cheek, the same as me. John calls it my 'beauty spot', and I wanted him to see that, too. Perhaps the lady was just a nice picture of myself after all.

Helping the lady? I felt guilty because they were my private stairs, and I was responsible. No one else was supposed to go down there. It seemed very, very important for me to get her back again.

John came in when I tried to stop him? I thought it was his fault that the lady had disappeared. All I wanted was to get her back up, but John started to come down too, and this made me angry.

Dark presence down the stairs? I think this was why I was shouting at John. I didn't want him to see whatever was there.

The boiler? We don't have a boiler or anything like that in the house, so it wasn't a real one. I do remember how my brother used to annoy me by referring to our mother as 'the boiler'. It was only fun, of course. I suppose he meant 'a tough old bird'! Perhaps that is where it came from in the dream. My mother was not in the dream. It is possible that I thought John might think of *me* as an 'old boiler', and I certainly would not like that.

Carrying a vase? I don't know why I wouldn't let John put his flowers in it. It was just that I felt it was my private vase, for *me* to put things in, and it should stay down the stairs, as though it had something to do with the 'boiler'.

Hit John with the flowers? I was angry, and then I felt sorry. There was no excuse for doing it in the dream. It was just temper. I suppose I *do* have a foul temper sometimes, but I don't want anyone to think of me like that.

Themes: Up-and-down emotions turning into sheer bad temper. Wanting to present one person, and hide another.

Conclusion: I suppose I want John to see me as a 'beautiful person' and not a bad-tempered 'tough old bird'. Well, who can blame me?

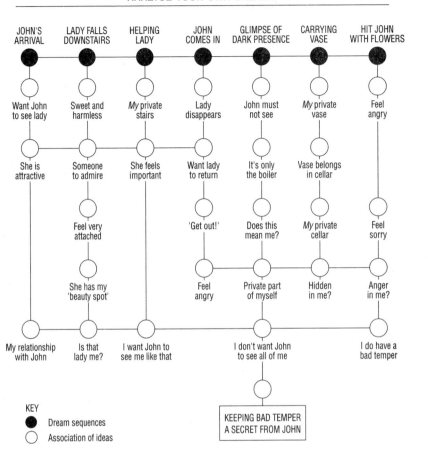

JOHN'S ARRIVAL	LADY FALLS DOWNSTAIRS	HELPING LADY	JOHN COMES IN	GLIMPSE OF DARK PRESENCE	CARRYING VASE	HIT JOHN WITH FLOWERS
Want John to see lady	Sweet and harmless	*My* private stairs	Lady disappears	John must not see	*My* private vase	Feel angry
She is attractive	Someone to admire	She feels important	Want lady to return	It's only the boiler	Vase belongs in cellar	
	Feel very attached		'Get out!'	Does this mean me?	*My* private cellar	Feel sorry
	She has my 'beauty spot'		Feel angry	Private part of myself	Hidden in me?	Anger in me?
My relationship with John	Is that lady me?	I want John to see me like that		I don't want John to see all of me		I do have a bad temper

KEEPING BAD TEMPER A SECRET FROM JOHN

KEY
● Dream sequences
○ Association of ideas

Later in the book it will become clear that the last example dream included the so-called persona and the shadow – both symbolic parts of the self. But for now it is important to believe in your own interpretation of your own dream, rather than a ready-made one couched in someone else's terms. Working on one's own dreams results in finding a personal source of wisdom, and the kind of guidance that comes from within, rather than from the outside.

Try not to be too logical about your interpretation. Your logical mind usually wants to keep your own 'story' acceptable to yourself and the people around you, and is liable to reject anything too new or unknown, unflattering, or not quite 'nice'. Don't play safe to the extent that you are misled by a comfortable but false interpretation. Dreams often involve factors which we have ignored or denied while

25

we were awake, and these are the factors that have been suppressed by our surface minds. These things need to be uncovered, understood and released if our analysis is to have real value.

WHEN SYMBOLS KEEP RECURRING

Chapter 6 should be helpful in giving you general ideas to consider about symbols. Recurrent dreams, involving the same symbols time and time again, are usually giving you a message about some problem that has been affecting your life in an unfortunate way – a problem that you don't like to look at in more realistic terms. Concentrate on these symbols and *feel* the emotions that their memory brings. Your *hidden* emotions, the inner feelings, are the source of dream imagery, and you will only understand the dream fully when your outer, everyday emotions are stirred too. The following is an example of a continually recurring dream:

> ℂ In this recurrent dream I am always looking through my wardrobe trying to find something suitable to wear. I know I have to hurry and go out to join in all the activity outside, but I just can't find any clothes that seem right. Everything is too shabby, or old-fashioned, or too brash, or the wrong size or colour. I get very anxious, wondering what to do.

This is a symbol-dream that really needs no analysis beyond simple acceptance of the symbol itself. As a dream symbol, clothes represent the way in which a person thinks of herself, or himself, and the way in which others think of them – or the way the dreamer *thinks* others think of them. This dream means that the dreamer has been lacking in self-confidence. Her own inner feelings are telling her that there is really no need for this. Never mind if her clothes – or her image – are not quite right for the occasion; she is wasting her potential by holding back all the time.

RELATIONSHIP DREAMS

The same symbol can symbolize a person, a place, a circumstance, an institution, or a principle, presenting an indeterminate number of meanings at one and the same time. As we have already seen, slang expressions can feature as symbols too – some kind of 'play on words' which, in the spirit of pantomime, make their appearance as real items in your dream. You may notice that women tend to dream in symbols more than men do. Men tend to build their dreams more around everyday experiences, giving them the appearance of real life; but they are no less dream images for that. They can still be hiding the truth within the fabric of a story. Unlike the collective symbols described in Chapter 6, personal dream images have symbolic validity for you relevant to your own experience, and they are likely to be known to you alone.

For living-together couples, the subject of male–female relationships tends to give rise to more dreams than anything else. Within a relationship, dreams can bring out a partner's deepest feelings better than the conscious, waking self. Both partners' egos will have been overruled, to help them see the situation as it really is. We all tend to build up artificial defences within any relationship involving give and take: we have our habitual little ways of disguising what we really feel, as the following example may show:

A WIFE'S DREAM

€ There was a tall tower, and I was peering through an opening into what looked like a dungeon at the base. Inside I could see some dead birds, and I'm not sure what else. My husband was standing behind me, and he asked me what I could see. I peered in again, and said: 'A dog's body.' My husband laughed and said, 'We'll soon clear it out!'

Tall tower? It was very strongly built. It makes me think of the saying, 'a tower of strength', and that makes me think of security, something firm and dependable – rather like marriage is supposed to be, or a family.
An opening? This was simply a convenient hole for me to look into, but various things had got in there. They were hidden things, and my husband was asking me what I could see in there. Perhaps he couldn't look in for himself. Perhaps it was only for me to look in.
Dungeon? I did feel in the dream that it was like a dungeon. Naturally, dungeons and towers make me think of being a prisoner, a princess held captive in a fairytale. But there was no princess in there, only dead creatures and assorted rubbish.
Dead birds? I suppose the birds had got in and couldn't get out again, though there seemed to be nothing to stop them flying out through the hole. Perhaps they had died and fallen down there. Dead birds make me think of lost hopes, lost freedom. Birds are so free to fly about. I remember feeling sad about it.

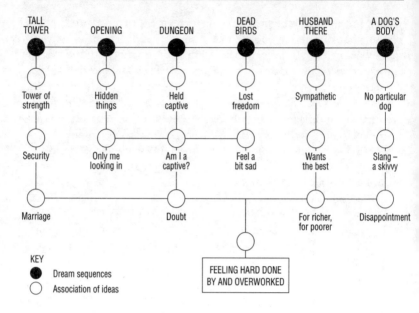

TALL TOWER	OPENING	DUNGEON	DEAD BIRDS	HUSBAND THERE	A DOG'S BODY
Tower of strength	Hidden things	Held captive	Lost freedom	Sympathetic	No particular dog
Security	Only me looking in	Am I a captive?	Feel a bit sad	Wants the best	Slang – a skivvy
Marriage		Doubt		For richer, for poorer	Disappointment

KEY

● Dream sequences

○ Association of ideas

FEELING HARD DONE BY AND OVERWORKED

Husband was there? He was being sympathetic and reassuring about the unpleasant things I could see. He meant well, and he didn't want me to have to look at nasty things. But it seemed that I was the only one who could actually see them. I could only tell him about them.

A dog's body? We have had a dog in the past, but this wasn't any particular one, just an anonymous dead dog – I think – lying among the birds. But in the dream I didn't say, 'A dead dog', I definitely said 'A dog's body', and I thought afterwards that this is a slang term for a skivvy, or a drudge, or a menial person who does all the work and no one cares about. I don't know what this has to do with me, really. We have a loving relationship and we both work hard together to make a go of our business. I hope it doesn't mean that I think I'm hard done by. That wouldn't be fair to my husband.

Theme: Frustrated hopes, vague disappointment, a feeling of being trapped and undervalued.

Conclusion: It does seem to have been a picture of our marriage and my doubts, my feeling of being trapped in a lot of hard dull work and the loss of freedom. This aspect of the partnership is a bit disappointing, though I know the business is doing quite well now, and we shall soon be in a much better position. I did marry 'for richer, for poorer', after all, and I think analysing and understanding this dream has perked me up a bit.

NOTE: They stayed together in a happy working relationship until the husband died in his eighties.

A HUSBAND'S DREAM

€ In my dream I was driving a bus with several passengers on board, including the wife. The wife was being difficult, and kept stopping the bus and getting off, trying to direct it. She tied a rope to the front axle and tried to pull it, and when that didn't work, she started pushing it about and rocking it from side to side quite violently. She was holding the journey up and making it difficult for everyone, and I was feeling quite exasperated, though in the dream I was trying to be patient.

Driving a bus? I am not really a bus driver, but in the dream it seemed to be my normal job. Everything would have gone smoothly if only the wife would sit down and enjoy the trip instead of making trouble.

Wife stopping the bus? She is never very patient at the best of times, and now she was determined to disrupt the journey. All I wanted was to carry out my job of driving the bus and carrying the passengers safely.

She tied a rope to the bus? I suppose she had to, if she wanted to make the bus go herself, because she can't drive, either in the dream or in real life.

Pushing and rocking the bus? It was doing no good at all. The bus was going nowhere, and it was uncomfortable for the passengers. I couldn't see any sense in it, but she was determined.

Feeling exasperated? Of course I was. Nobody was getting anything out of it, she was gaining nothing, and we were getting nowhere. If she wanted to try and drive the bus properly, she could; I wasn't stopping her.

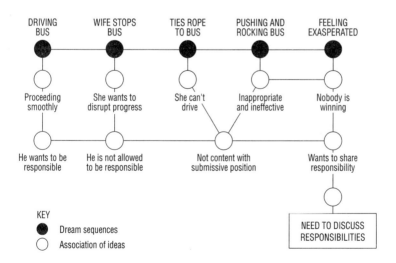

29

Theme: Unreasonable behaviour, incomprehension, lack of co-operation, clash of desires and responsibilities.

Conclusion: I know it was only a dream-bus, but I do like to take my responsibilities fairly seriously. I don't think I want to be 'head of the household' in particular; I'm not bossy. But having thought about this dream, it seems that the wife feels discontent with the present situation, and will not let me persevere with my present course. It all seems to boil down to making a better job of sharing responsibilities.

NOTE: They stayed together for a few more years, and finally separated, though still on friendly terms.

WHEN YOU HAVE A BAFFLING DREAM

You can analyse most of your dreams in the way set out in this chapter. But occasionally you will experience a dream that defies analysis; one that seems perhaps to have great urgency, and yet no personal meaning, in terms of your own experience. You may be sure that it does in fact have great significance for you – if only you can grasp its meaning! When this happens you may suspect that your own little dream has somehow become superimposed on or mixed up with a much larger, impersonal type of dream. The ensuing chapters will touch on dreams of this sort; experiencing and trying to understand them will set you on an adventurous voyage of the mind. It may even take you further than the mind can travel unaided: a journey to infinity.

THREE

THE WORLD DREAM

ALL THAT WE SEE OR SEEM
IS BUT A DREAM WITHIN A DREAM.

Edgar Allan Poe

*T*HE human body is made of solid bone, flesh and blood; the world on which we live is a solid sphere of rock, its tidal oceans stocked with life forms, its dry land clothed for the most part with vegetation and also inhabited by living creatures of solid bone, flesh and blood. All these are material forms. But once we have started to take an interest in our dreams, we quickly learn to see through solid flesh to the non-material self we know to be there.

To take the matter further, we can learn to see through the solid materiality of the world itself. Our dream life will be greatly enriched, and our understanding of it infinitely enhanced, when we are able to do this. We will become aware of a new dimension in dream awareness when we can see the world of nature itself in the form of a dream – the dreaming state of world consciousness – and express that state as a background to our dreams. When I first began to record my dreams, this was one of the earliest:

There was bare stony clay; then I saw that it was a termites' nest, with convoluted tunnels, towers and shafts; then I saw that it was a great city, with tall buildings and churches, and people hurrying about; then gradually I became aware that it was all a vast sleeping female figure who stirred in her sleep. I knew that this was the great earth mother, and that she was dreaming.

This dream expresses a first inkling that solid materiality may not really be quite so solid and lifeless as it seems. The collective memory of the great world dream is still part of ourselves at a very deep level, to be recalled occasionally in our own personal dreams. It gives us a glimpse of the natural world in its subtle, non-material state. The trappings of civilization are solid and heavy, and they tend to hold down our inner awareness which would like to explore such things. We are made to feel somehow guilty for entertaining such abstract thoughts, for even our thoughts seem to cycle around materiality – things chasing yet more things endlessly, throughout our lives.

Once we know what it *is*, we can well imagine that, in uncivilized days when people still lived close to nature, and when manufactured objects were virtually non-existent, the great world dream was closer to human awareness. The Aborigines of Australia still refer to the state

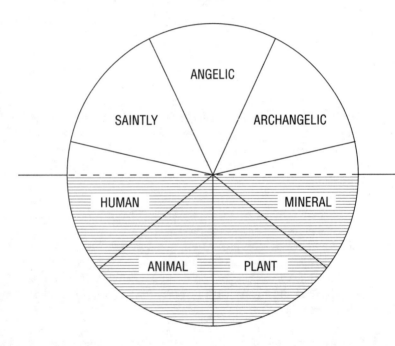

The world mandala. The world as we know it is symbolized as lying in darkness below the horizon: the great 'world dream', gradually evolving from chaos and bare rock, through the slow development of plant and animal life, to human understanding and the dawn of awakening.

of Dreamtime to explain their own origin – their emergence from world consciousness through the mysterious 'dreaming' process of nature.

The imagery used to express these ideas will vary from race to race and from country to country, of course; our dream images tend to relate to our own previous ideas and experiences. But we can all make use of the same mandala principle as an aid to understanding. The mandala this time will represent the whole world in its non-material form, rather than an individual person. If the personal, dreaming self can encompass the whole collective pool of humanity in its imagery – and we have seen, or will soon see, that it can – it can also embrace the whole world in this subtle sense, and experience it as a series of dream images.

WE ARE NOT SAINTS

Forget the restrictions of logic. Try to visualize a mandala expressing your own personal self, superimposed on a full-scale world mandala. As before, the horizon will bisect the circle; everything above this line is visualized as being in the daylight; everything below as belonging to the night. Above the horizon now are the higher degrees of awareness, or conscious attainment, all of which are normally far beyond the human condition, and unapproachable by us. Below the horizon is the familiar world of nature and material things, and this is where we live.

Visualize this mandala now as representing the whole human race, as well as you, the individual, and as well as the world itself. On the left of this mandala, the physical human sector is partly in the light at its highest point, the symbolic point of sunrise and new birth. This illuminated portion represents the extent to which earth-bound yet non-materially orientated humans can experience the world of spirit by becoming saintly people. But, of course, very few of us are saints.

At the other end of the horizon, at sunset, and the symbolic point of death, the mineral or material sector also extends upwards into the light. This shows the extent to which the vast majority of materially orientated people can become aware of the world of spirituality, through their own desires. You could identify this illuminated section on the right of the mandala as 'the light of the occult'. People in between the two extremes, including those who are orientated towards their own sensuous (animal) and aggressive (plant) natures, either in their dreams or in their daily lives, remain wholly in the dark as far as spiritual matters are concerned.

As before, a natural cycling process is at work. We have already considered the possibility of personal 'wholeness' – and I believe that our dreams illuminate the slow but steady movement towards that ideal end. We should all be experiencing an inward momentum carrying our own psychic centre of gravity through the underworld of nature, from the 'material' to the 'human' zones. Our own conscious awareness, we must remember, is now below the horizon, rather than above it. The aim of the world dream is to wake up into the light of dawn, and in this scale there is no way a person can ascend from the material or 'mineral' sector to the bright 'archangelic' state above it; the cycling movement runs in the opposite direction. The only way we can wake from the world dream, to come to full awareness, is to pass through the 'human' sector into the 'saintly' sector immediately above it.

ONE THING YOU *CAN'T* DO YOURSELF

If you think this is an entirely obscure and abstract piece of reasoning that has nothing to do with our everyday lives, you are quite wrong! Whenever we have the idea of reaching a 'higher state', of achieving some kind of immortality through our own efforts, or of contacting the 'spirit world', it means we are clinging to the material end of the spectrum. Work, career, worldly responsibilities, all these are of a material nature and need our best efforts; but the one thing you *can't* do for yourself is to reach a higher level on the spiritual plane. People who suppose that spiritual answers are to be found through science and learning are themselves to be found in the farthest regions of the material sector too, basking in the light of their own erudition.

It is a seductive situation that extends far beyond an individual's dream-life, but dreams will provide a clue and a timely warning. The idea of submitting your own will to a higher, divine will may sound naïve and old-fashioned to many; but the simple act of heeding the warning and accepting the message, adopting 'the humble part', does result in travelling *with* the world dream, rather than following the crowd. The principle often appears in our personal dreams, expressed as an alternative course of action, or an unpopular choice.

☾ I dreamed I was on a busy street with everybody heading for the bright lights of town. My friends were walking along arm in arm, laughing and joking, and I wanted to join them. Near a shop there was a car parked on the pavement, sort of backed against some bushes in the dark. I wanted to tell someone to move the car as it was in the way. Then I saw that it was concealing an old signpost pointing along a path leading out of town. The path went a very long way through the trees and a park with horses and deer. I heard one of my friends say, 'Come on! You don't want to go that way!' But I knew I had to see what was at the end of the path.

The dream certainly did relate personally to the dreamer and her friends, and the fact that she had been worried about getting into trouble with the law. But the background to her personal dream was the world dream itself – seen as a conflict between the things that most people want, with the pleasure they get out of them, and the gentle influence of the world cycle, the counter-flowing current of dreams. The dreamer did not actually *want* to follow the lonely path through the trees; it was something that she felt she ought to do.

CLIMBING TO HEAVEN?

If in your dream there seems to be a strong element of *wanting* to climb, *wanting* to follow some path, this too can be a gentle warning that this particular path is not the right one for you. Dream imagery is infinitely variable, and what in one personal dream may be seen as a busy street leading to the bright lights of town may, in another, seem like a direct route to heaven itself. Your own dream will let you know, through your feelings, whether it reflects a course of life that is running with the world dream, or against it.

❡ At the start of this dream, I found myself with very many more people, going along a high ridge, so narrow that we had to crawl in case we fell off. We seemed to be creeping along the knife-edged top of a mountain ridge. We could just see that on one side it was grass-covered and almost perpendicular. We couldn't see the other side as it seemed to be straight down from underneath the narrow path. Gradually the people in front of me seemed to have disappeared, and I was then in the lead. Then I heard giggling and laughing behind me, so very carefully I turned my head and saw three boys (round about fourteen years of age) who were laughing. One of them said, 'Shall we tell her?' But one of the others said, 'No, let her find out for herself.' They then got over on to the grassy side, and slid rapidly out of sight. I went carefully on, then realized there was no longer a grassy side. In fact, there was nothing under the path where I was. I could see that a tremendously long way down there was a sort of very pleasant-looking parkland, where a lot of people were walking about. The path I was on came to an abrupt end. It was impossible for me to turn round so I started to edge my way backwards. This was very difficult and nerve-racking. At last I caught a glimpse of grass; but as I looked it just seemed to move further back. This happened again and again. I got into such a panic that it woke me up.

This dream is connected with another dream recorded in the final chapter. It was experienced by an elderly widow who had already dreamed that her late husband was climbing up a steep place – so she assumed – towards heaven. She had been trying to re-establish contact with him in one way or another, and this was the lesson taught by the dream: her conscious aim had been to rejoin her husband by following him on the climb, but when this sort of decision is made deliberately, as the world dream explains, it is bound to lead only to the heights of materiality. The world dream teaches us that the only dream-climb, the only spiritual journey that can be truly rewarding on a long-term basis should follow the direction of the natural cycle, leading from the state of materiality where most people live (and rightfully so), back through the dark world of nature to the point of human birth, or rebirth. If you are religious, you may recognize parallels in your own religion. For Christians, 'to become again like a little child' is essential before you can enter the realm of saints.

WHAT THIS MEANS FOR YOU

Can you avoid trying to travel in the wrong direction? Certainly you can! Simply remember your dreams and accept their message. And in your waking life, if ever you feel the urge to control non-material affairs, to attain some sort of higher state, or to contact the spirit world, or to rise above the common herd in some way, forget that urge. Simply remember that there is a greater will than yours, and agree inside yourself to be carried along by that will. Whether you have a religion which you follow, or not, your hopes will be realized in the very best way, because you will be in harmony with the world dream, and thence with the whole of creation.

Look again at the mandala diagrams in Chapter 1. The world mandala (page 32) is rather like a photographic negative of the personal mandala: in the personal mandala our conscious part is limited to the upper half, which is filled with light; our unconscious part occupies the lower half, which is filled with darkness. In the world mandala, virtu-ally all of us live only in the lower, dark half. Creatures of nature (and in this sense, that includes us) are quite unaware of world conscious-ness, or the bright dome of spirituality above them. Nature is the world's sleeping and dreaming process at work. In this sense we, along with the lives of animals, plants, and even minerals, mountains and rivers, are all merely dreams of the non-material world — of the great earth mother.

In the light are the worlds of what we call the saints, the angels and the archangels. If you wonder why it should be like this, and why the archangelic light apparently shines down into the material sector (known by Jews, Christians and Muslims as the satanic power), you need to look towards mythological stories of creation for the answer. Science is not much help here, for science itself belongs to materiality, and cannot venture outside its material limits. Perhaps the principle is best expressed in poetic terms, as it was in the seventeenth century by the blind poet John Milton, in *Paradise Lost*, describing the fall of the Archangel Lucifer:

> Him the Almighty Power
> Hurled headlong flaming from th' ethereal sky
> With hideous ruin and combustion down
> To bottomless perdition, there to dwell . . .

In the symbolism of the great world dream, the Archangel Lucifer was obliged to become the adversary, Satan, to rule in the zone of materi-ality.

> Is this the region, this the soil, the clime,
> Said then the lost Archangel, this the seat
> That we must change for Heav'n, this mournful gloom
> For that celestial light?

The sensation of falling often features in unpleasant dreams, and usu-ally occurs at the evening-end of the night, soon after dropping asleep. The dream itself will very likely have a counterpart, some sort of related experience in waking life that triggered the dream, and which can be analysed by the dreamer. But this is its root: the great fall mir-rored from the world dream; the inevitable plunge from the brilliance of world consciousness down to the darkness of materiality. Sometimes it is no more than a brief sensation; there are many forms which this basic dream can assume, but this example is perhaps typical:

> ℂ I was on the battlements of a church tower, and decided to climb up to the top of a pinnacle to see the view from there. Then a robed figure like a bishop came clambering on the wall towards me, and said, 'It's not safe. Wait till the builder's been!' But I said, 'I don't care about that!' And the next thing I knew I slipped and was falling in panic. I woke up in a sweat.

DAWN DREAMS OF THE WORLD

So the sensation of falling is related to the thoughts and impressions of the day passing down into the subconscious at night, but on a world scale. But what will the dawn dreams of the world be like – the vivid, re-created outcome of this vast dreaming process? I think we all know the answer; but because the principles involved are non-material, the idea can only be expressed in symbolic terms, in the imagery of dreams. The wide-awake, fully conscious world is basking in the light – the light, we must assume, of divine wisdom – while the creations of nature live darkly within the world of dreams; it is only by way of the dawn dreams of the world that we as human beings might one day come to whole awareness – the perfect consequence of materiality.

This vast 'unconscious' mind of the world, formulating the impressions gathered during its spiritual day, collates and develops them by way of the growth of plants rooted in the soil, through the mobile and more actively conscious lives of the animals, through the yet more conscious but still dark and primitive stirrings of humanity. Through the entire gamut of the natural world, finally arriving at lucid awareness in the sunrise of the whole assimilated human self. This is the perfect outcome of the world dream: the evolution of nature, culminating in the perfection of the human psyche.

Because the mandala covers our own personal life as well as the collective life of the world, we can readily appreciate that these sectors within the world of nature can equally be seen as sectors of our own nature: a human part, an animal part, a plant part and a material part. Of these, the material part is the most solid and tangible – not merely our material bodies (for of course we are all material objects in that sense), but our psychic contents as well, the subtle, world dream nature of materiality.

MATERIAL FOUNDATION OF DREAMS

Can there be such a thing as subtle materiality, or are these two contradictory terms? To arrive at the answer, let your mind dwell on the characteristics of minerals, of any material body, any bunch of atoms. Materiality includes the force of gravity, magnetic fields, and all the laws of physics. Gravity has a 'need' to gather everything into the deepest, heaviest part of itself, and hold it all together; a 'black hole' in space has this nature. When translated into human terms, intellectually and emotionally, this 'need' signifies 'greed', the desire to possess, to have and to hold. The concept of materiality as an essential foundation for human life is a constantly recurring background to our dreams:

€ In my dream I was in a place like the Grand Canyon, or an enormous quarry. There were miners or quarrymen far below me, digging out 'heavy metal' and carrying it along the bottom of the canyon towards some factories. Factory smoke was blowing up the canyon. I was going to climb down when I met my family sitting on some rocks. They were moving their heads and talking and smiling at me, but then I saw that their bodies seemed to be made of stone growing out of the ground. There were lots of very pretty little stones piled up round about. I looked at some of these stones admiringly. Then mother got up and said, 'They may look very nice, but what use are they?' and she closed the door. Then I saw that we were in our house.

This was an unformulated dream remembered when the dreamer woke up early in the night after sleeping for an hour or two. It expresses how completely dependent we are on the material instinct. Even our own bodies are material objects, and we could not live without it. It ensures that everything falls into place and functions correctly, according to physical laws. But there is not really any sense of altruism in it, of helping or caring. When children grow into adults they seem to become filled with this type of instinct, and feel the need to acquire all sorts of things for themselves – money, houses, other people as partners or children, or employees, consumer goods of all sorts; all the good things of life. Nobody is to blame for this; we live in a material world and it is good to share in its bounty.

THE SPIRIT OF SCROOGE

It is the basic material instinct that persuades some people to become misers, hoarding gold and gloating over it, dismissing kindness and generosity as mere weakness. In his famous story *A Christmas Carol*, Charles Dickens created everybody's archetype of the miser with his character Scrooge. Scrooge has a dream in which he sees the ghost of his late partner, Marley, so loaded with the chains of materiality that he cannot rise from torment. He is shown visions of his own past, present, and possible future unlamented demise, if he does not alter his attitude towards life, and his fellow human beings. This is a great literary example of an instinctive, creative dream, possibly drawn from Dickens's own personal unconscious, yet based upon the world dream: a glimpse of subtle materiality, when this has been allowed to fill the self to the exclusion of higher possibilities.

Do not think that psychic materiality, or materialism, is something that only affects misers. In the main, 'materially orientated' people are just the ordinary, normal people with whom we come into daily contact. As an acquired part of the whole human instinct, materiality is quite essential for civilization: it enables us to make and use tools, clothes, buildings, vehicles, and all the other useful things we have come to rely upon. Also, of course, it is the source of weapons, from thrown stones and spears to bows and arrows, to Kalashnikovs, rocket missiles and hydrogen bombs.

So material characteristics are somewhat contradictory: they are wholly normal and socially acceptable, friendly even; and yet at the same time they are blindly destructive and totally uncaring. Dreams, of course, are not themselves material entities. 'Material' dreams, or in this sense 'evening dreams', simply reflect the essence, or the nature, of materiality. As they represent merely the start of the world dream process – the evolution from bare rock and water through plants and animals and humans, to the highest superhuman possibilities – these infant dreams themselves will tend to be unformulated and unresolved. They may quite likely be of a destructive or dangerous nature. They may provide the inspiration for new inventions, or they may equally well reflect the trivial and the mundane, the uninspiring and the obscure.

HARMONY WITHIN THE WORLD DREAM

Some dreams illustrate or log the dreamer's inner progress when he or she does seem to be living in harmony with the steady cycle of the world dream. One or two dreams of this sort will be featured in the final chapter, but an example will be useful here, if only to show how closely some people's dream imagery corresponds with the nature-categories of the world mandala – progressing from the mineral, to the plant, to the animal, and to the human sectors.

☽ I was walking in the dark but carrying a lead-light such as I use at work – an electric light bulb on a long lead trailing behind me. I was walking along a path with bushy, overgrown vegetation on either side. Then I came to an open field, and I felt the lead plug jerk out of its socket, having reached its full extent, and the light went out. There were sheep in the field, and I walked among them in the dark. Then the path came to a place where I couldn't go any further, and I stopped. But looking ahead, I saw myself still walking on, along a road lit with street lamps.

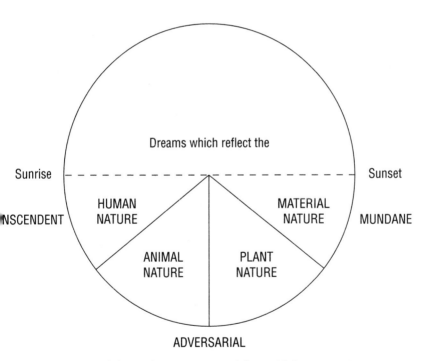

Our personal dreams bear an imprint of the world dream, varying or progressing through the night as though to reflect the hidden nature of earth's life forms.

This dream very clearly expresses the progress of the dreamer's life journey, running with the flow of the world dream. Plants are rooted in the earth. In effect, the dreamer within any sector has something of the inner nature of that sector: the individual whose psychic centre of gravity is within the 'plant' sector is also still rooted – still dependent upon and closely attached to materiality. The light lead becoming unplugged as the dreamer left the bushy vegetation and reached the open field where the sheep were grazing means that this psychic connection with the material force had been severed. The dreamer's psyche, by way of the inner feelings, moves through the 'animal' sector, and on reaching its limits – his current position in life – is still able to see ahead, to see his future self on the 'human' road.

In Chapter 1 we saw how personal dreams may change their nature according to the hour of dreaming – depending upon how far the dreaming process has developed through the individual's sleeping time. The same thing applies to individual dreams based on the world dream, for the life-zones of plants and animals contain something of the nature of the shadow, on a grand scale. Like the shadow of the subconscious mind, these dark contents of the world dream may emerge in the form of an unexpected adversary, or a hidden danger. On the face of it we may expect certain animals to act in a dangerous manner, but at first sight plants do not seem particularly threatening, or likely to frighten anyone – until we take a world-scale view of their fiercely competitive lives.

THE SECRET LIFE OF PLANTS

From the plant's point of view, within the world dream, humans seem to live their lives at a frantic pace. From the human point of view, in waking life, plants seem to live their lives in slow motion. But they too have instinctive movements, triggered by light, gravity, moisture, air, touch, and the need to feed. If these were speeded up, we would see that plants are constantly on the alert, waging war with each other, struggling to the death without let-up. It is as if each individual plant possessed an inbuilt drive to take over the world, which it pursues to the limits of its own individual nature.

€ In my dream I was walking in a dense forest with sunlight filtering through the crowns of the trees. Everything near the ground was dark and mysterious. Instead of green, everything round about was red, or black, but this did not seem at all unusual to me. The ground was squelchy and sticky, as though saturated with blood. All around I sensed great danger lurking in the darkness, and I seemed to *feel* a great roaring and shrieking, rather than *hear* any actual noise. The tension seemed unbearable. I knew there was a way out of this forest not far away, where everything would be much safer, and I tried to press on towards it, but felt as if I was rooted to the spot, and could move only very slowly, as if wading through treacle. Perhaps it was the blood holding me back.

The dream provides a vivid if frightening picture of the plant world – part of the world dream in which an individual person has somehow become involved. It is not surprising that the predominant colour is red, rather than green. Remember that on this scale the dream is like a negative transparency – in this case a colour negative – of a personal human dream. Green is seen as red, its opposite and complementary colour. Plants thrive in an infra-red environment, for this is the light of their hidden inner world. It is the dream of someone who has in some ways turned his back on materiality, on the rat-race of materialism. But, like an intruder in a fairytale, he really has no right to be in that dream forest. If he could have analysed his own dream (see Chapter 2) it would probably have a personal meaning for the dreamer. He felt trapped in his own turbulent thoughts and desperately needed a way out of his problems; but this does not alter the fact that the images are on a world scale, tapped directly from the unconscious mind of the world itself.

How does this dream-world forest compare with its counterpart in real life? Imagine a great forest, or even a friendly little bluebell dingle by the brook. If a tree dies of old age, or is blown down in a gale, a great number of infant trees – offspring of the dead tree and those surrounding it – will crowd into the gap and struggle to compete with each other and grow upwards to find a place in the sun. They also have to compete with the ground vegetation which, in turn, engages in a frantic race to take best advantage of the opportunity for life. Above the ground vegetation the understorey of bushes and shrubs also put on growth in the struggle to get their heads above the others, roots probing for any available feeding space. Some of these plants are able to live humbly beneath the shadow of taller neighbours, until the shade becomes too dense. Others find it impossible to survive any cover at all, but must battle to reach the light quickly, or die.

So, from the viewpoint of the world dream, the woods are not such a peaceful place: they are gory battlefields, filled with the victorious, the defeated, the dead and the dying. Ancient forests may seem stable communities – but only because all the members are constantly at daggers drawn with their neighbours, defending the place which they have won. Even the welfare of their own children counts for nothing. You will see that dreams dominated by the plant sector of the world's unconscious mind will tend to have the nature of aggressive competition, of ruthlessness, or deeply rooted hostility.

THE SECRET LIFE OF ANIMALS

As we move on through time, through the earth-night, through the evolutionary process, life-forms become detached from the earth: animals of course are rootless and free-ranging. They too can be hostile and aggressive, but their hostility is largely territorial, competitive, and full of bluff, involving a battle of wits rather than the ruthless suppression of one another that is typical of plants. If they kill, it is a one-off affair of necessity. No hostility is involved in killing another animal merely to eat; this is the mechanics of the continuous cycle of nature, a dream within the world dream.

Frequently involving pride tinged with wariness and ever-present sexual desires, dreams using symbolism of the secret world of animals can carry important lessons regarding social interaction. Moral boundaries are often a matter for the animal rather than the human nature. Animals normally have and maintain strict rules governing their own behaviour and that of others of their species, and do not care to breach them. This is basic morality: being true to one's instinctive barriers and boundaries.

Rules are important to the unconscious mind, and breaches of instinctive rules are frequently at the root of adversarial dreams. Such dreams will probably not involve animals at all. However, I frequently hear about dreams in which the dreamer seems actually to be an animal, involved in specific animal pursuits. These dreams too may bear a personal message for the dreamer when analysed, but taken at their face value alone, they can offer an intriguing view of instinctive animal life. The dream that follows was in fact analysed in terms of everyday life, and did have something important to say to the dreamer about her family relationships, which there is no need to go into here.

€ In the dream I was a fox – a vixen – and I was searching around trying to find my cubs, when I saw sitting in some very long grass a large dog fox that I was very anxious to get away from. So I jumped a

44

nearby hedge on to the road, and crossed to the other side, then went on down the road for a short distance, then started to cross back again. About half-way over, a large bus came round the bend above me at speed. I only just had time to reach the side and jump the hedge. The ground here went down very steeply towards what I recognize now as the Cotswold village of Broadway. When I had woken up, I wondered why I had been so afraid of the dog fox. Another peculiarity was that there seemed to be no colours in the dream; everything was in varying shades of grey.

THE HUMAN ELEMENT

We all think of ourselves as intrinsically 'human', to match our physical bodies, our brains, our emotions. But the evidence of our dreams shows that, for the most part, we seem to be centred in the less-than-human sectors of the world mandala. Even the most intellectual, the most distinguished, the most pious of us may turn out to be more at home spiritually in the worlds of animals, or plants, or material objects, than in the human category. It is a good job we are not given to worrying about it, or it would certainly drive us mad! People whose centre of gravity is actually within the 'human' sector may not *seem* to be better people. They may in fact be less clever, less moral, less well regarded than those who are firmly centred in the apparently lower categories of life within the world dream.

Boundaries and limits can more easily become blurred in the world of humans than in the corresponding worlds of plants, animals and things. This is because humans are freer than the lower creatures of nature – we have the choice which they lack, and it is this choice which enables the world dream to be brought to a worthwhile conclusion. People seldom dream directly about their situation in the world mandala – unless they are currently changing, have risen to a more evolved station in life, or are in danger of sinking to a lower one. To dream that you have left a lower condition and reached a higher one is always good news, though its message may be disguised:

> I was on a chain bridge over a river, looking back at some jungly forest full of fierce animals. The animals could not walk on the chains. There were creatures in the river too, but they could not survive out of the water. I was quite relieved to cross the river and reach the village. A friendly dog ran to greet me, but then I saw it wasn't a dog, but a boy I knew. I said, 'I thought you were a dog,' and he laughed.

Then I was in a market place, full of people and stalls with meat and fruit and vegetables, and birds in cages. The people were a very mixed bunch: white people, black people, Chinese and Arabs, and lots of children.

In the context of this chapter, in the light of the world dream, the deeper meaning of this dream seems fairly obvious. Outside of that context, without the world mandala as a base, its imagery is fairly cryptic. The dreamer had been going through a sticky patch at work, and felt very deeply that it was 'a jungle out there'! Wild animals seemed an apt simile for his colleagues, clients and nagging employers, and he had decided to leave his job to try self-employment in the travel industry. Naturally it had been a worrying time for him, and the future still seemed uncertain. But when the world dream reference was pointed out to him, his self-esteem and confidence received a much-needed boost. When a person returns to human status, in this sense, by remembering his or her own dreams and submitting to the world dream, the real-life move from employment to self-employment is a step that fits the new-found independence and freedom of choice.

WORKING TOWARDS 'BUDDHA CONSCIOUSNESS'

Please don't imagine that this great cycle, the world dream of nature, is something quite apart from the ordinary dreams which you may find yourself remembering and recording. It is always there, as a kind of backdrop to all our petty hopes and fears, and the basic source of dream imagery. Your dreams of everyday relationships, uncertainties and problems, may not display dramatic imagery. But from your own observations you may discover that, when your dream shows you possible solutions to your problems, the nature of these solutions will vary according to the time when the dream occurred. It is sure to correspond with one of the categories of the natural world, and the instinctive passions associated with them. Thus, evening or early-night dreams are likely to provide unfeeling or even destructive attitudes; later in the night, your dreams are likely to display angry, highly emotional and aggressive reactions. Later still they may provide a more reasonable answer to a problem, but one which is likely to provide for your family or personal group at the expense of outsiders. Dawn dreams are likely to point to the most constructive, the most truly 'human' conclusions.

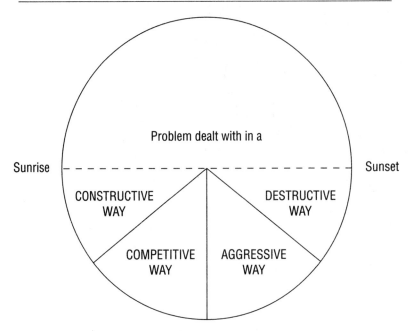

Problem dealt with in a

Sunrise ———————————————————— Sunset

CONSTRUCTIVE
WAY

DESTRUCTIVE
WAY

COMPETITIVE
WAY

AGGRESSIVE
WAY

The nature of dreams tends to vary according to the hour of waking.
Worries and problems that have been on our mind during the day may
be reformulated in a way that reflects the underlying nature respectively
of minerals, plants, animals and humans.

There is a continually growing or maturing process at work in the unconscious mind on a world scale, and this is reflected in the personal unconscious: as above, so below. The world dream develops from bare earth and stone, in which life-forms take root and develop, becoming more evolved until they somehow pull their anchoring roots loose and roam the earth as beasts, which evolve in their turn until they become humans. Human understanding could be said to have grown from animal instincts, destined eventually to reach the zone of spiritual light, or world consciousness. It will then be able to share in the broader scale of awareness that has been called 'Buddha consciousness', when the human sphere matches and coincides with that of the earth itself. This is one aspect, one explanation of the symbolic state of wholeness towards which our dreams are working.

THE PSYCHOANALYTICAL APPROACH

IF WE MEDITATE ON A DREAM SUFFICIENTLY LONG AND
THOROUGHLY – IF WE TAKE IT ABOUT WITH US AND TURN IT
OVER AND OVER – SOMETHING ALMOST ALWAYS COMES OF IT.

Carl Gustav Jung

WE have much to owe the Big Three – Freud, Adler and Jung – for their combined work on formulating the unconscious mind. For all generations previously, 'unconscious mind' would have seemed a contradiction in terms, for 'unconscious' implies negation of the quality of conscious awareness implied by 'mind'. The term 'psyche' came to be used in preference to 'mind', for it can more easily embrace the notion that part of the human mind – perhaps the greater part – operates on a level beneath that of conscious awareness. Without this breakthrough, this basic division of the mandala into light and dark, conscious and unconscious, our knowledge of dreams would be no further advanced than that of the ancients – and ancient assumptions about the process of dreaming were as many and as varied as the ancient cultures themselves.

The Big Three, of course, were medical psychologists, and the dreams they heard about were mainly those of people suffering from psychological problems of one sort or another – those people who appeared in their consulting rooms. But as Jung might have said (and probably did), 'We are *all* neurotic'; we are *all* influenced in what we say and do and think by our own unconscious contents, which have been building up in us since birth, and probably, it seems, before that.

As far as the process of dreaming is concerned, there is no difference, either in symbolic substance or formative material, between psychiatric patients and the rest of humankind. The psychoanalysts simply acknowledged that dreams offered the most convenient way into the abstract territory of the unconscious mind, and that a study of dreams might allow us to glimpse something of the mysterious processes at work. When they interpreted their patients' dreams, the psychoanalysts were searching for possible causes of neuroses. We are studying dreams in a more general way, not so that we can point triumphantly at the root of a problem, a trigger-point, but because we are intrigued, and we want to learn the language of dreams.

The psychoanalysts at least partially rejected the artificial mind-bending methods that had become popular at that time (and which, sadly, have become popular again): the use of drugs and hypnosis, under the influence of which the individual, not being fully in command, is unable to come to decisions and understandings on his or her own account. They were keen exponents of the do-it-yourself principle, acknowledging that only the individual personally concerned could satisfactorily explore all that goes on in the darker recesses of his or her own psyche. This is a voyage of discovery that can bring about a new dimension of being, an experience of newly found confidence that does not involve merely the earth-bound materialistic ego. It takes courage to explore honestly your own subconscious mind, let alone the vast expanse and unfathomable depths of the collective unconscious. Cleverness of mind, they acknowledged, is seldom the key to success in this field. Excessive cleverness, being limited to surface awareness, tends to boost the ego, and often attempts to concrete over the uncontrolled, unclever parts of the psyche – the unflattering parts that have been 'thrown away' into that rubbish pit in the backyard of the mind.

HUNGRY FOR SEX

We might be excused for thinking that Freud seemed to be somewhat obsessed with sex. He saw dreams as yet another expression of repressed sexual desire. He conceded that there may be an occasional dream with no sexual content, but even then, he claimed, there will be a sexual element which has become so distorted by the dreaming process that it is no longer recognizable as such. It was that distortion that represented the great barrier, the resistance set up within the self to prevent conscious exploration of the unconscious mind. 'We desire most that which is forbidden,' he said, and as sexual desires are usually

49

the most forbidden or the most taboo factors in our society, they are the factors that tend to become repressed. Not only do we dread others knowing our contents in this regard, we even dread the possibility of knowing about them, of rediscovering them, ourselves. In his view, dreams reflect neuroses, and neuroses occur because we are all hungry for sex, but usually pretend not to be. Repressed sexual desire, he claimed, is the chief factor at work in the subconscious from early childhood on, forming our character and moulding our behaviour.

Freud referred to those desires of the self which tend to become repressed as the *id*; these dark desires, he said, were opposed by conscience – by what he called the super-ego. The id seeks only gratification, has no morals, and is driven by basic instincts – but these basic instincts mean that it may display human judgement, and can be selective in working towards long-term benefits. It is that part of us that demands attention and seeks selfish expression. The super-ego he saw as an artificial self which builds itself up and strengthens itself during our lives, and people filled with it are liable to become over-inflated, or self-important. Some people are mainly 'id'; others are mainly 'super-ego'. Running between these two extremes is a flow of psychic energy Freud called the libido – desire – and he saw this flow of energy as directed principally towards sexual gratification. In this he differed from his colleagues Adler and Jung, who ascribed a more general interpretation to the aims of the libido, considering it to relate to other facets of personality besides sex.

Freud was referring to everybody, and not merely his patients, when he claimed that all our psychological quirks can be traced back to some childhood experience, to some trauma or series of unfortunate events that our conscious minds have forgotten. Such events will have caused a fixation, a psychological hiccup that brought back the childish attitude – quite appropriate at the time of the event – to recur in adult life, and make itself known whenever a similar event occurred; whenever the subconscious memory of that old trauma was triggered off. In men, he identified what he termed the Oedipus complex: boy children came to hate their father for robbing them of their mother's love. When they were old enough to understand the reasons for this, the guilt they felt formed the basis of the super-ego. Girl children displayed what he termed the Electra complex: coming to love their father and hating their mother for similar reasons, and with similar results. Most people think that Freud's theories were too narrow, that the sexual contents of our minds, though powerful, are not quite so all-devouring as he claimed; and even he diluted his theories somewhat in later years.

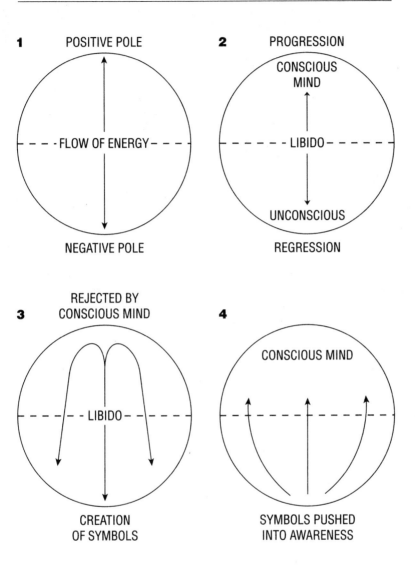

The psychoanalysts' understanding of the way dreams are formed. Freud, Adler and Jung ascribed varying properties to the libido – but, as a flow of energy alternating between positive and negative poles, its principle remains the same in each case. Any instinctual drive that is rejected by consciousness will be returned to the unconscious mind, where it becomes transformed into dream images.

DREAMS AS CARTOONS

By what process does material that has been rejected, for any reason, by the conscious mind become converted into symbols, and emerge as dreams? Freud believed that the psyche includes a built-in censor, whose function it is to disguise the form of anything which the conscious mind finds distasteful. He termed this centre the 'endo-psychic censor', visualizing it as a psychic force able to modify anything incompatible with the dreamer's conscious self-opinion. In effect, it is able to produce a cartoon picture out of a real situation, making it less offensive and thus more acceptable to the waking mind. The purpose of this psychic centre is to allow the dreamer to find mental expression of and some relief from all these repressed longings. He noticed that a dreamer might relate a dream enthusiastically, and find it amusing or even flattering; but if he or she realized the real message of the dream, they would probably feel mortified. You can understand the significance of a political cartoon in the newspaper only if you know something about the people and events to which it refers. Without this knowledge, it will be merely an amusing drawing.

Freud divided the actual contents of the dream into two types: the manifest, and the latent. The manifest content sets the scene with details taken from the dreamer's own waking experiences. The latent content is the plot of the play – the cryptic political message of the cartoon, and the true meaning of the dream. The following example dream was recorded in 1997, but I think it is one that Freud could well have been told about in 1897:

> ℭ In the dream I was lying on my stomach on a hill, looking at a hole like a rabbit burrow. A creature poked its snout out; it was pink and quivering. I put an arm down the hole and pulled it out. It seemed to have some sort of nectar on it which looked very nice, and I kissed it. Then a large polecat-like animal ran down the hill and caught the creature and started to shake it. Suddenly the polecat turned into a schoolmaster whom I knew, and the pink creature escaped and ran away down the hill. I said: 'No, I'm not chasing after it. I'm not bothered at all!' The schoolmaster pushed his face into mine very angrily, but I just laughed at him. Then I started to feel sorry and uneasy.

Freud, I am sure, would have seen this as an Oedipus dream, full of sexual images. The young man who dreamed it, he would have said, is recalling his own babyhood in his mother's arms, in the context of all his experiences since then. It suggests infantile memories of the nipple, while the animal characters in the dream reflect the nature of the passions involved, and the moral implications which it hides. The stern father-figure is angry, demanding his conjugal rights and overruling the overtones of latent infantile sexuality – only to be rejected by his own son and, later, to be the cause of guilty feelings.

THE WILL TO POWER

Where Freud put the psychic accent on sexual impulses, Adler put the emphasis on an inner drive for power. He saw the inbuilt need for self-assertion as the basic motivation of people in general, and of young people in particular. Indeed, we could truthfully say that the approaches of both Freud and Adler are likely to appeal more to young people than to the middle-aged and older categories. Once people are old and experienced enough to have a fair idea of who and what they are, and where they want to go, they will probably find that the ideas formulated by Jung hold the most appeal for them – not as a matter of intellectual choice so much as emotional satisfaction, of what seems to fit in with their own feelings, their own instincts, and their own long-term ambitions. An old person's long-term ambitions, after all, are not limited to the rat-race of this world.

On one thing the Big Three were agreed: that if the great reservoir of unconscious, repressed material within the self could be recovered and reassimilated by the conscious mind, the individual would as a result be better adjusted as a person; they were also agreed that dreams offered a convenient and effective way into this inner world, the better to examine some of those contents. But where Freud saw sexual desire as the main seat of neurosis and the main substance of repressed material, Adler identified the drive for power as the most important factor, and psychological problems he saw as childish attempts to compensate for a basic sense of inferiority. Adler held that children in particular are bound to suffer from feelings of inadequacy during their first five years of life, being small and weak and uninformed, and he saw the resultant inferiority complex as the common root of individual faults, of personality defects, besides the substance of dreams.

Everyone, Adler argued, possesses a will to power, and if this will is frustrated the individual is bound to look for ways in which the balance can be redressed. He or she will seek gratification by hook or by crook; if his or her practical accomplishments are not successful enough to achieve coveted self-confidence, the individual tends to fall back on fantasy and pretence. Feelings of inferiority cry out for compensation, he said, and people who suffer from them are liable to try to dominate other people, and circumstances, in any way they can. They are likely to be difficult in company and refuse to co-operate with those they regard as more fortunate. But this basic feeling of inferiority can also have the positive effect of encouraging people to achieve, to excel at anything that might attract the admiration of the world in general, and win praise from those closest to them. This basic drive, Adler claimed, is reflected in our dreams too.

We behave in our dreams, said Adler, in the way we would like to behave in real life; dreams in effect are emotional rehearsals, during which we can practise and perfect modes of behaviour that will make us seem more admirable, more praiseworthy, more powerful than we know or suspect ourselves actually to be. Dreams, he thought, show up our stumbling-blocks, our petty fears, everything that causes us to hesitate in social situations when we ought by rights to be asserting ourselves in a more positive way. The warnings and encouragements transmitted by dreams are aimed at showing us how to surmount those obstacles which stand in the way of our personal supremacy.

New growth in the desert

And so Adler saw the craving for power and status as the basic, if hidden, obsession that influences our lives from early childhood on. But if and when that craving for power becomes satisfied, he would probably have agreed, it will give way to the sexual drive, to the craving for sexual success. According to Adler's theory, power is the dominant theme during the first five years of life, and this is the period during which our attitudes are fixed, our neuroses rooted. But quite soon after that age, the phenomenon of puberty starts to happen, and the will to sex takes over as the dominant theme. In this regard, we could say that power progresses to sex, that Adler's system gives way to Freud's, as though part of a natural cyclic process.

We are back on more familiar territory now: if we set this idea of psychic progress against the world mandala – the world dream – the pattern reveals itself. From the spiritual lifelessness of the material sector, the psychoanalytic movement has set the cycle in motion. There is a grander life hidden within the recesses of the mind. Dreams are not after all merely manifestations of our repressed sexuality and our cravings for power. They match the inner workings of the world dream itself. From barren rock and desert, plants eventually grow, and seek power as a first priority, to assert authority over other plants and claim their own piece of desert. The following example is a typically 'Adlerian' dream:

> ⓔ I seemed to be struggling through a deserted, barren place without any sign of life. There was plenty of abandoned rubbish, old cars and petrol drums and heaps of builders' rubble. Apart from these it was like the Sahara, with loose sand difficult to walk in. I felt uncomfortable and weak. Then I came up to a huge stone wall. It seemed to be a fort like you might see in films about the Foreign Legion, or the Crusades, and I tried to get inside. There did not seem to be any way I could get in, or climb up the wall. There were a few people on the battlements, walking past and ignoring me, and I started to shout and wail. Some of them glanced down at me with contempt, and then went about their business. I felt very small and helpless.

This was the dream of a man who had been going through a difficult time at work. He thought of himself as ambitious, but could not seem to progress or make any impression on his employer. He did not get on very well with his colleagues, and felt that his employer was a bully who wanted to keep him in a menial position, and would not give him the chance he deserved. He was toying with the idea of starting out on his own, but was rather afraid to take the first plunge into the unknown. The dream fits into the world mandala in this context: to a plant a lifeless desert represents an utter lack of power. There would seem to be no reason, in terms of space and opportunity, why a person – or a plant – should not succeed, without limits, and yet it does not and cannot happen. The situation is barren and hopeless, and seems little better than death.

Adler's system is certainly one step, or one world-sector, ahead of the materialistic view that sees dreams only in terms of wanting, hoping and fearing, wish-fulfilment, or disappointment. But many people even today overlook the discovery that dreams, at root, are organized by an intelligence that is distinct from individual content: an intelligence that takes into account not only the needs of the individual most concerned, but those of everybody else in a position to help the process along, as well. Perhaps the Big Three have taught us, besides their valuable theories, that over-specialization may result in overlooking the broad view, and that dreams, like neuroses, can take many different forms.

A COLLECTIVE INTELLIGENCE

If you study 'dreamworkers' as well as dreams, it may soon become obvious that people who take an obsessive, and particularly a professional interest in dreams tend to concentrate on the type of dream most appropriate for them – naturally enough, for these are the ones they experience for themselves; the dreams that correspond with their own position in terms of the world dream, their home-sector within the world mandala. The Big Three set the pattern:

Freud takes his place in the middle; sex, for him, is at the centre of everything, and without it no creature could exist. Adler takes his place on one side of this central position; Jung moves to the other side. By the nature of their work, they represent individual striving to attain

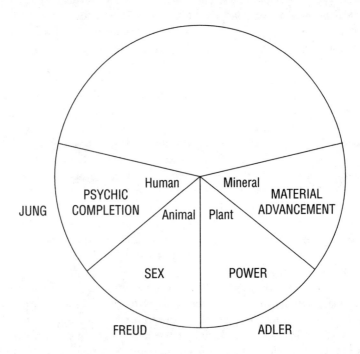

This diagram can be superimposed on the world mandala (page 32).
It suggests that psychoanalytical processes halt and reverse 'progress',
or the common drive towards material advancement, regressing by way
of personal 'compensation' as formulated by Adler, through Freud's
view of sex as a driving force, to Jung's theory of 'individuation'
leading to psychic completion.

a higher, a more coherent state; their 'patients' were people who found the material world a disturbing place in which to live. The bulk of the human race are materially orientated, and 'live' in the mineral, material zone: material advancement dominates their inner awareness. They represent the unformulated, 'evening' dreams of the world.

As a result of this, if you buy a dreamwork manual, the chances are you will find it full of examples of material dreams, and material interpretations. Most people's dreams seem to be locked within that world sector, the material zone of the world mandala. Everything 'human' within that zone, whether a waking impression or a dream, has to be explained in terms of the outer personality, through the workings of the everyday, personal mind.

The world mandala drops the hint that all dreams originating below Jung's point of entry are less than truly human. Even though the dream imagery will take human form, it will have the essence of material objects, of plants, or of animals. Dreams, like people, need to progress, to mature, to follow the subtle movement of the world dream. We do not, of course, need to become psychiatric patients in order to make this happen. Only truly human dreams relate to the collective unconscious, which is filled only with non-material images, not of nature, but of humanity. Spiritual dreams start here too, for the human world of spirit is intimately associated with the sea of the collective unconscious.

How can our dreams be changed from a concern with material advancement to a concern with psychic completion? This is what needs to happen if we are to follow the drift of the world dream and achieve the goal of the self. On a personal scale, it is well known that dreams can be induced and then directed by hypnotic suggestion, in such a way that the hypnotist can decide both the subject and the outcome of the dream being experienced by suggestible subjects. On waking, the dreamer will relate what the hypnotist wanted to hear, and already knew. If an individual hypnotist can do this, what happens when the far greater collective intelligence takes a hand? Freud's 'endo-psychic censor' no longer selects images to mollify the waking mind. When our dreams come under the supervision of the collective intelligence, they will contain material from beyond the dreamer's waking experience. They may also be selected to involve and inform other individuals as well.

When I started reading Jung's work on dreams, in the mid-1960s, my partner (who had no concept whatsoever of Jung) obligingly began dreaming and relating vividly explicit dreams full of 'Jungian' symbols, which I was able to interpret with confidence. It seemed plain that those dreams had somehow been formulated and produced especially for that reason: so that *both of us* could learn from them. Since then I have seen it happen again and again: dream imagery produced as required to serve current needs, not merely on a personal basis, and not by any personal intention. It seems that a single collective intelligence is at work behind the scenes, a universal 'endo-psychic censor' capable of guiding us all.

ARCHETYPES OF THE COLLECTIVE UNCONSCIOUS

Jung was powerfully aware of this collective dimension in a way that Freud and Adler were not. Jung could see a tendency common to all, enabling modern people to understand life in a manner psychologically conditioned by the past history of mankind – a tendency which he called archetypal. Archetypes, he said, are shared forms of apprehension which probably existed even before the development of consciousness as we know it: inborn conditions of intuition, or 'primordial images', which could take the form of unquestioned emotional certainties, or of dream images. They reach the surface of awareness notably on important occasions: birth, death, danger, triumph, defeat, during changes of psychological orientation such as puberty, or any unfamiliar, awe-inspiring or frightening experience. Unconsciously, when such things occur, we still use the imagery of our ancient ancestors – those ancients who were not yet familiar with the world of materiality; people who in spiritual terms were still close to their own innocent childhood.

The most common archetypes include: in men, the anima, or female soul, and in women, the animus, or male soul – which enable the two sexes to understand intuitively the other's very different point of view; their advice can help the man to be sympathetic, and the woman to be assertive, when the occasion demands. Other archetypes include the king, or wise old man, who always has good advice to offer; the great earth mother, or goddess, who can provide similar (if more earthy) advice; the persona – the social mask people tend to wear; the shadow, which adopts an unlimited variety of forms and with which we are already familiar; and the self, often seen as an innocent child observing the world. The body of these figures may be formed, or 'filled in', by the dreamer's own life experiences, but their essence is primordial and archetypal.

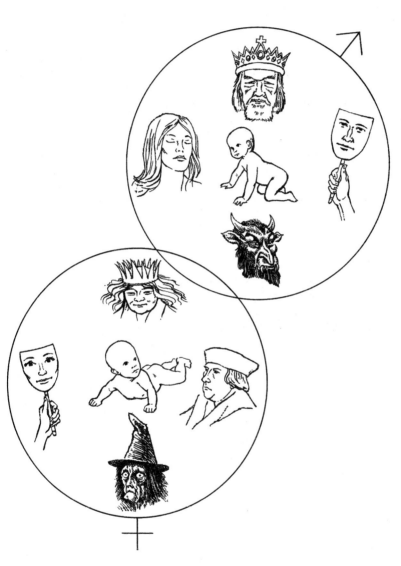

Archetypes of the collective unconscious. In a man: the child self; the king (a wise man); the anima (a chaste maiden); the shadow; and the male persona. In a woman: the child self; the goddess (or great earth mother); the animus (a father-adviser); the shadow; and the female persona.

59

ANCIENT MYTHS

Jung claimed that in dreams people often experience archetypal symbols to be found in the myths of ancient civilizations – matters about which they had no conscious knowledge. While pointing these features out, he believed that people should try to work things out for themselves, and find the meaning of their own dreams, taking a broader and far less dogmatic view than either Freud or Adler. He encouraged the people who consulted him to draw or paint their own dreams, recording them like an illustrated story, to bring out the symbolism while the memory was still fresh. This is still an excellent exercise which will encourage further meaningful dreams of this sort. To portray your dreams in this way sets the self on a course sympathetic with the world dream. The following dream example seems to me one that could well have been related to Jung. Simple enough in itself, it is full of ancient symbolism:

> ☾ I was walking through a forest and came upon a sunlit glade, in the middle of which was an old stone column with a sundial on top. I went up to it, and saw it had writing on it which said: 'Time is Joy.' There was something like a banked ditch all round the sundial, with ivy growing in and along it. I parted the ivy with my hands and looked through it, and glimpsed ancient ruins and carved stones. In the ditch it seemed I could see to a great depth with many different layers, and there were people and horned animals of some sort. Then I saw nuts rolling on the ground, and looked up to see, standing by the sundial, a tall bearded man wearing a robe. He had a kind, gentle face, and was carrying a baby who was chuckling, and holding out a nut.

Jung would no doubt have pointed out several connections with ancient myths in this dream. Ivy, as well as the vine, is a symbol of Bacchus, or of Dionysus, a god of the earth, who belongs equally to the world below and to the world above. He has often been represented in myth as a robed, bearded man with a kind face. Dionysus was identified with Faunus, and with Pan, and with Silvanus, all spirits of the forest who let the future be known in dreams. He was also identified with Kronos, the god of time and change. This ambivalent figure can also represent the dreamer's archetypal father figure, or a wise old man who can see the future. The chuckling child is none other than the dreamer's self, being carried willingly along by this kind and gentle power. Nuts in ancient times were used as playthings, like marbles, or as pieces in throwing and gambling games. Nuts too are full of hidden meanings – they can represent the head with its concealed thoughts, or potential growth hidden in the future; the eventual fruiting of the forest of the mind. The celebrations over which these gods of growth presided, involving horned animals, were joyful occasions, something in the nature of a present-day harvest festival. The stone column of the sundial, by its phallic shape, represents generative power; the sundial itself is a personal mandala, with everything that such a symbol entails. All these themes are interlinked, and express the renewed workings of an ancient process of personal fulfilment.

THE DREAM WORKSHOPS APPROACH

LET'S CONSIDER WHO IT WAS THAT DREAMED IT ALL . . .
IT *MUST* HAVE BEEN EITHER ME OR THE RED KING. HE WAS
PART OF MY DREAM, OF COURSE – BUT THEN I WAS PART
OF HIS DREAM, TOO!

Lewis Carroll, *Through the Looking Glass*

*J*F you like the idea of sharing your dreams and dream interpretations, the dream workshops approach may be the right one for you. Lone wolves are do-it-yourselfers. The shared approach may seem more suitable for gregarious, outgoing, socially interactive people. Everybody tends to dream dreams that reflect their emotional lives, and in particular their relationships with others. If you lead a particularly busy, active life, your subconscious may have become gorged with half-digested impressions. Filled with unformulated and unresolved problems, the memories of your dreams may seem like a confused, tangled web of interlinking events and social relationships. If this is the case, if you are suffering from 'dream indigestion', it may be right for you to seek out a dream-worker, or fellow dreamers who will help you to unravel your dreams and reach a constructive conclusion.

DIRTY LINEN

Bear in mind, however, that dreams sometimes contain hidden layers of meaning which, when analysed, may reveal unpleasant or unflattering matters that many people would find too personal, maybe even too embarrassing, to share. Your psychic underwear may be pulled out of the laundry basket and spread out for all to see and gossip about. So, if you do not like the idea of this happening, I would suggest that the do-it-yourself method is best for you.

Not a few people, though, simply love to wash their dirty linen in public, and to discuss their emotional and sexual problems in detail; some of the free-and-easy audience participation shows on TV will bear this out. Who is to say who is right? If you like to talk about yourself – and if so you will certainly be in the majority – well, why not? And why should others not get to hear about it? Understanding your dreams on a shared basis will do much to allay emotions that are flying out of control. The fact that you are sharing your problems can reassure your worried mind, and can ease relationships that have become strained. Your social life will probably become more pleasant as a result, for this is the area of life within which dream workshops analysis will have the greatest effect. After that initial step to set you on the right track, it will be up to you to climb the dream mountain alone.

Sharing your dreams with others will help you to look inside your own mind, help you to discover and assimilate your own brand of hidden wisdom, to find your own key. You may have been baffled by a dream – perhaps because it was confusingly complicated; or possibly because it was misleadingly simple. The do-it-yourself method described in Chapter 2 may not seem to have produced the hoped-for results, and in this case, allowing someone else to prompt your thoughts with a few appropriate questions will often help. That other person may introduce a viewpoint that had not occurred to you; you will have found a new stance, a new way of looking at an old problem. The guided conclusion of the following example dream was an eye-opener for the young man who dreamed it:

¢ In my dream I had gone to visit 'the old home'. It was a large mansion which had obviously seen better times, and had plainly been neglected for many years for it looked on the point of falling down. It had gables and ornate little towers that looked unsafe. It had slates missing off the roof, the porches were crumbling, the woodwork was rotted, and the staircases were rickety; all the plaster was falling away, the windows were broken and the shutters hanging loose on their hinges. I had intended going back to stay for a while, but as it was plainly an uninhabitable ruin, I did not go inside.

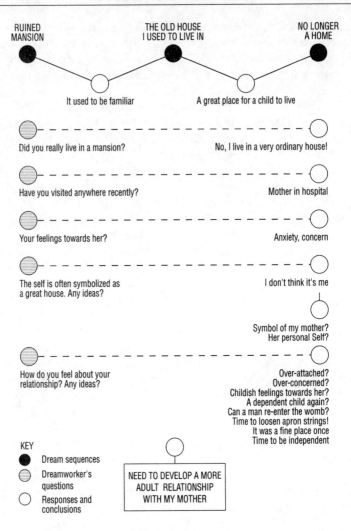

PASSIVE AND ACTIVE ROLES

This last example was a completely passive dream which contained a hidden psychological truth. Its assimilation set the individual concerned on a new course through life, though the dreamer did nothing in the dream except to observe the old house. When you first start remembering and recording your dreams, your own role in them does tend to be passive – you are merely watching while the dream takes place before your sleeping eyes. But as time goes by, your dreaming self tends to take a more active part in the dream. Instead of remaining a member of the audience, you will have become an actor, playing your own role, acting and reacting with the other dream characters. Dreamwork has tended to confirm that the way we act in our dreams – whether in an active, reactive or passive role, reflects the way we habitually behave in real life. Assimilating the message of your own dreams can have a positive effect on the sort of person you are.

Being passive is not quite the same as possessing a gentle nature. It sometimes happens that people who live very quiet, inoffensive lives may find themselves dreaming violent dreams, full of aggression and passion. Or the situation may be reversed: a person who is hyperactive in real life may experience dreams of peace and beauty, and restful pursuits. This is only to be expected, as your dream-life works towards wholeness and balance. Ideally, we should all possess an even balance between action and inaction. We should be assertive when the situation calls for control, submissive when matters cannot be controlled and must therefore be tolerated. 'Balancing dreams' are often concerned with morality: excessively moral people may dream of letting their hair down; wild ones may dream of piety and prudence. Dreams which are discussed or even acted out in company – some dreamworkers recommend staging a little play of your dreams with fellow dreamers – may help to make these issues clear by pointing out inner discrepancies and balancing the outer personality.

SEEKING COMPENSATION

Sexual compensation is sometimes demanded by the physical body when deprived of its natural function. This may emerge via the inner feelings, in exaggerated imagery by way of dreams. I recall the case of a devout Muslim who, having committed himself to a complete ban on sex or licentious thoughts during the fasting month of Ramadan, dreamed he was having enjoyable sex with the Imam – his prayer leader. On waking, he was utterly devastated by such apparent wickedness on his own part, and, unaware of his own unconscious contents, became convinced that he was being taken over by an evil spirit.

Dream sex may be making a point to the conscious mind, indicating that repression is taking place, or that resentment for some reason is building up to reinforce the shadow. The inner feelings, unlike the everyday emotions, are able to take the long-term view; better to shock the waking conscience than to create a monster in the shades of

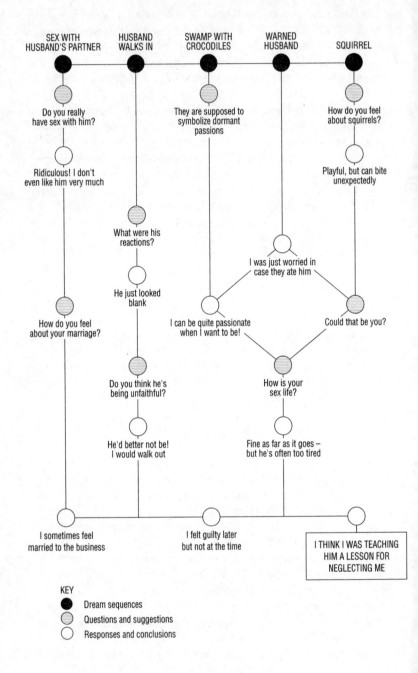

SEX WITH
HUSBAND'S PARTNER

HUSBAND
WALKS IN

SWAMP WITH
CROCODILES

WARNED
HUSBAND

SQUIRREL

Do you really
have sex with him?

They are supposed to
symbolize dormant
passions

How do you feel
about squirrels?

Ridiculous! I don't
even like him very much

Playful, but can bite
unexpectedly

What were his
reactions?

I was just worried in
case they ate him

He just looked
blank

How do you feel
about your marriage?

I can be quite passionate
when I want to be!

Could that be you?

Do you think he's
being unfaithful?

How is your
sex life?

He'd better not be!
I would walk out

Fine as far as it goes –
but he's often too tired

I sometimes feel
married to the business

I felt guilty later
but not at the time

I THINK I WAS TEACHING
HIM A LESSON FOR
NEGLECTING ME

KEY

● Dream sequences
◐ Questions and suggestions
○ Responses and conclusions

66

the subconscious mind. The following example also came as a shock to the dreamer, this time a married woman and devoted spouse.

> ℂ I dreamed that I was lying in bed, having sex with my husband's business partner, and was just reaching a glorious climax when my husband came into the room. I nodded and smiled at him, and he started to walk up to me, but I think there were some crocodiles in a swamp at the side of the bed, and I warned him not to step on them and stir them up, as they might be dangerous! There was a squirrel sitting on one of the crocodiles' back, and it sprang on to the bedrail, chattering. Then I woke up, feeling quite elated.

Through various questions and suggestions, the fellow dreamers in her group helped her to arrive at a satisfying conclusion, though it did little to ease her long-term feeling of frustration.

BREAKING THE RULES

The personal unconscious is the natural home of morality and law-keeping. Look back at the world dream, and you will recall the natural origins of morality, of observing boundaries, of following the rules of your own species – in our case the human race. Our conscious minds may allow us to do things that we would certainly refrain from doing if someone in authority were watching – breaking the rules in small ways. On the surface we may think this is perfectly acceptable, if we can get away with it. But under the surface of consciousness we can get very upset by this sort of behaviour, without even realizing it! This state of affairs features quite often in dreams, and it may need a few gentle questions to uncover the truth. The result, if it is accepted, will be a better-balanced psyche.

> ℂ I was in a sort of room lined with hundreds of different shapes of all different colours. There was a narrow space between some sort of cupboards, with some people outside. To show them how easily I could get through this narrow gap I held my arms above my head and sort of danced through. Then I saw that I had touched the sides, and picked up a nasty stain on my blouse.

Perhaps it was the inconsequential event of 'shopping' during the previous day that triggered off this rule-breaking dream. Such triggering events frequently provide a clue to the interpretation of your dream.

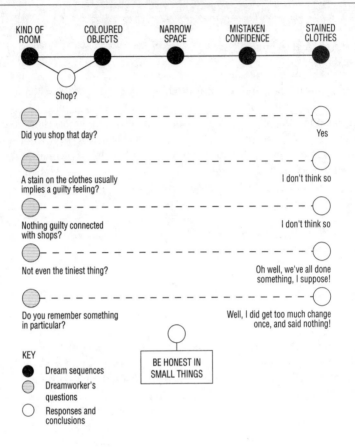

KIND OF ROOM   COLOURED OBJECTS   NARROW SPACE   MISTAKEN CONFIDENCE   STAINED CLOTHES

Shop?

Did you shop that day?   Yes

A stain on the clothes usually implies a guilty feeling?   I don't think so

Nothing guilty connected with shops?   I don't think so

Not even the tiniest thing?   Oh well, we've all done something, I suppose!

Do you remember something in particular?   Well, I did get too much change once, and said nothing!

BE HONEST IN SMALL THINGS

KEY
● Dream sequences
◉ Dreamworker's questions
○ Responses and conclusions

It is always advisable to write down your dream as soon as you wake, if it helps you to remember it. But remember to resist the temptation to embroider the details, to alter the fabric slightly to make it seem more interesting, or to show yourself in a better light. You are more likely to succumb, perhaps, if you are following the workshops approach, because you will be aware that the details of your dream are likely to be shared. Make sure they are the true details!

Shared or not, make a point of recalling and writing down any real-life events that you think could be even vaguely connected with the subject matter of the dream. Your unconscious mind recognizes associations with past events, and may be using them to tell you something. Some long-repressed emotional hurt which would be better aired and resolved – this is the type of thing at the root of dreams, triggered by recent incidents and categorized as similar by the subconscious.

RE-ENTERING YOUR DREAM

Try to re-experience and re-enter a dream that seems to you to have been unfinished. You need to sit somewhere quietly, make yourself comfortable, and close your eyes – but don't go fully to sleep. Recall your dream gently. Do not try to think around it; simply re-enter it, and let the sequence run through by itself. You should be re-experiencing the dreaming state without actually sleeping. Follow the dream step by step; let it run on past its previous conclusion. As you are not really asleep, you cannot really 'wake up' when the dream is finished; allow it to continue until it reaches a satisfactory conclusion. Do not permit yourself to become sidetracked, and avoid deliberately inventing incidents or solutions – allow the sequence to unfold itself naturally.

In a dream workshops situation there will probably be someone to help you, perhaps by getting you to describe every now and again what is happening in your re-entered dream. This will keep you on the right track, and encourage your own inner feelings to recall the spirit of the original dream, and bring it to its natural conclusion. By re-experiencing your dream in this way you will not have falsified it; you will have allowed it to be completed. The following example records an unfinished dream, the experience of re-entry, and its final outcome:

> ℭ I was in a place with several rooms joining on to one another, all fairly full of people, talking and laughing in little groups as though they were at a party. I was wondering which group of people to join. But then I went into another room, and there was nobody in there except a 'snorter', and I came out again quickly . . . I have no idea what a 'snorter' is, and I didn't actually see it. When I woke up I felt quite upset, but didn't know why. I was quite depressed for some time afterwards.

During the re-entry process the dreamer saw that the mysterious horror in the empty room was just an old coat; then the coat disappeared, and there was a girl whom she knew, and who was cold and crying. She said she felt sorry because this girl was on her own; she cuddled her, and felt happy to be with her. Then she explained that the lonely girl suffered from some sort of breathing difficulty like asthma, and was not very sociable. Having allowed the dream to reach its conclusion, she feels very much more understanding and friendly towards the other girl.

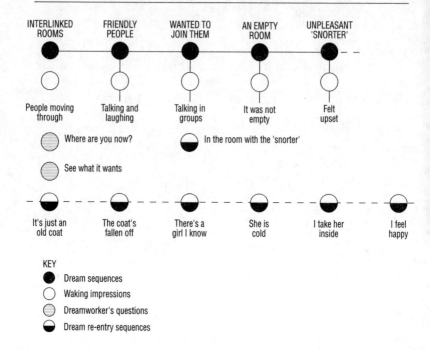

POWER AND CONTROL

'Personal power' and 'inner power' are seductive ideas, and very popular in today's high-powered world. However, we have seen that any conscious striving for inner control tends to create a movement counter to the natural flow of the world dream. Personal power, in this sense, leads the self back from the possibility of psychic wholeness and possible spiritual expansion, towards greater material strength. This may be fine for your body, and even for your status in the world – we all need physical, financial, material strength – but it is not the true destiny of the self. Our dreams show us that. It is not the ultimate goal of the dreaming process. Self cannot find completion in this direction; the self cannot be made concrete. For this reason it is best to forget the aim of 'power' and 'control' where your dreams are concerned. Most dream images, it is true, are products of your own unconscious mind; but if there is a lesson to be learnt through dreams, we have to submit our outer selves, and our will, to that inner message and all that it entails. It can be of no value to us to attempt to control it or dictate to it.

It sometimes happens that, when we are dreaming, our conscious ego intervenes and we become aware that it is 'only a dream'. Then, if we do not wake up straight away, we may find that we are able to manipulate the dream characters and direct the dream events. This is known as lucid dreaming. Some people recommend it, for it certainly works towards that popular egoistic principle of acquiring power in your life – of the feeling that you should be able to influence events and people, and to supervise your own subconscious processes. But by helping your ego to achieve this questionable power, your dream will have lost its originally intended purpose – that of making a point important for your whole psychic development. The pupil has to submit to the teacher, otherwise there will no longer be a lesson worth learning. It will have become simply an exercise in teacher-control by the pupil. In the following example the dream became lucid when the dreamer disliked the way events seemed to be going.

❦ I was inside a half-empty industrial building, looking around. It was important that I should not be seen or heard. I went up some stairs and into an empty room which I inspected, thinking in terms of how I could make best use of it. It had a heavy wooden planked floor,

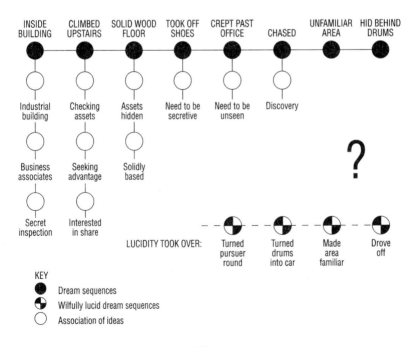

INSIDE BUILDING	CLIMBED UPSTAIRS	SOLID WOOD FLOOR	TOOK OFF SHOES	CREPT PAST OFFICE	CHASED	UNFAMILIAR AREA	HID BEHIND DRUMS
Industrial building	Checking assets	Assets hidden	Need to be secretive	Need to be unseen	Discovery		
Business associates	Seeking advantage	Solidly based				**?**	
Secret inspection	Interested in share						

LUCIDITY TOOK OVER: Turned pursuer round — Turned drums into car — Made area familiar — Drove off

KEY
● Dream sequences
◑ Wilfully lucid dream sequences
○ Association of ideas

71

grimy with industry. Then I heard someone moving on the floor above so I took my shoes off to walk more quietly, and tiptoed out of the room down the stairs. I slipped out of the building past the office, which was occupied, trying not to be seen, but someone saw me and came out. I ran away and they ran after me. The surroundings were unfamiliar, and I didn't know the best direction to run. I hid round the corner of a building behind a pile of empty drums or scrap metal. At this point I realized I was dreaming and decided to alter the dream. Almost like a puppet-master I made my pursuer turn round and run the other way. Then I conjured up my own car out of the old drums, made the street look familiar to me, and drove off.

A TRIP TO NOWHERE

You will see that a dream of this sort is not being allowed to arrive at its own rightful conclusion. The dream-cycle is being short-circuited at the crucial point. Instead of the inner feelings selecting and presenting a sequence of images, the everyday ego, realizing that it is being 'fooled', takes over control. The dream itself from that point on will be designed solely to please the ego – the source of power-feeling; your dream story will have become an ego-trip. Your psychic clutch will start to slip, and your vehicle of the self will fail to make progress, though the engine may be racing. This is not how it will seem to your mind. Your ego, and thence your self-confidence, will have received a boost; you may even have lost your fear of the unknown. But you are unlikely to meet the unknown part of yourself; you will merely gain the comfortable ability to manipulate your own imagination.

The same sort of thing happens involuntarily during a so-called wish-fulfilment dream, in which you dream that your dreams have come true! A condemned man may dream of a reprieve that never in fact arrives; a starving person will dream of food; a traveller lost in the desert and dying of thirst will dream of cool streams, or a glass of ice-cold water. Their powerful desires have forced an entry into the closed territory of their subconscious mind, and influenced the outcome of their developing dreams. A wish-fulfilment dream, as a waking memory, can masquerade as a truly predictive dream of the future, but in fact it is an ego-trip to nowhere. The following is a typical example:

ℂ As a student having just sat my final exams, I was worried about the results, as I knew I could have done much better. I dreamed that the results had come up, and I approached them with dread. One of the lecturers was there, and I said: 'Have I failed?' And he said: 'Failed? No! You've passed with honours!' The actual results came through a few days later, and in fact I had scraped a very ordinary pass.

ACCEPT THE MESSAGE

It would be odd if we did not wish to regulate our own lives, and to improve our own fate; but at this level within the psyche our power is limited. If you recall the world dream, you will realize exactly where the attractive idea of psychic power is coming from, and that it is likely to lead to a dead end. If you deliberately modify your dream, say, when a frightening situation occurs, you are refusing to accept the inner message.

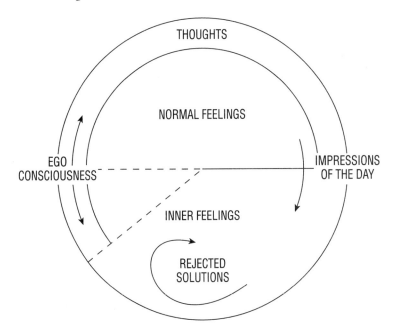

What happens when your dreams become lucid — when you realize you are dreaming — and consciously alter the way the dream is going? In effect, the ego is intruding where it has no right to be, rejecting the conclusion reached by the inner feelings. The natural balancing-out process of your dream will have been short-circuited.

73

The workshops approach – sharing your dream by relating it to others and listening to their suggestions – can help to avoid squandering your dream opportunities. When a dream starts to become lucid, when you become aware that you are asleep and dreaming, remember that you can use the opportunity to the good. The dream will be a vivid one. It may well happen that an unpleasant or frightening situation is developing, but try to experience it with patient acceptance: do not change it for something more pleasant; do not abandon it by waking up. If you do either of these things the problem will remain unresolved; the solution which is being formulated by your inner feelings will be lost. Remember instead to remain asleep and to continue with the dream, and to await the outcome with trust and patience. Always allow your dreams to resolve themselves naturally if you can, without interference from the ego, from your own desires. Allow your dream to be the teacher!

The example that follows is of a dream that became lucid, and in which the dreamer persevered under frightening circumstances:

> ℂ I dreamed that I was asleep in bed, and couldn't move. I was trying to get up and out of bed, but was completely paralysed. I was not alone in the bed, because next to me was a large wolf. I believe that (in the dream) it was someone's pet. I felt very frightened, first because I could not move, and second because I was aware that wolves are liable to attack someone when they sense they are afraid. This made me all the more frightened, because if the wolf started to bite me I couldn't escape. By this time I realized I was asleep and *dreaming* that I was trying to wake up. But then I decided to relax and just carry on dreaming, though I was genuinely frightened. The wolf did bite me as I had feared – on the legs. Then I realized that the bites had allowed the 'venom' that had paralysed me to run out, and this killed the wolf. After that I felt perfectly free to move, though I felt rather sorry for the wolf, which was only following its instincts.

The dreamer's predicament was rather like 'Catch-22', where either of the alternative courses of action depended on the other being completed first. The dream was also related to the world dream, and could be interpreted with that in mind. But the dreamer related it to a real and unpleasant situation at work, where she was being harassed by a fellow worker. The moral of the dream was 'give him enough rope and he'll hang himself', and she followed the dream's advice. She allowed the bully to have his own way at the crucial time, and the real-

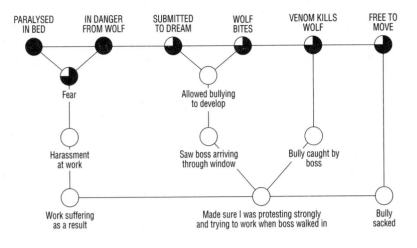

PARALYSED IN BED · IN DANGER FROM WOLF · SUBMITTED TO DREAM · WOLF BITES · VENOM KILLS WOLF · FREE TO MOVE

Fear

Allowed bullying to develop

Harassment at work

Saw boss arriving through window

Bully caught by boss

Work suffering as a result

Made sure I was protesting strongly and trying to work when boss walked in

Bully sacked

KEY
- ● Dream sequences
- ◑ Submissively lucid dream sequences
- ○ Real-life connections

life situation was reversed: the bully was sacked and the dreamer promoted. The dream is also unusual in that it uses the common and rather frightening phenomenon of 'sleep paralysis' to help make a point. The dreamer could have deliberately changed the circumstances of the unpleasant dream when it became lucid, but chose not to. Through heeding a little practical 'workshop' advice about dreams in general, the dreamer had allowed her personal dream message to come to reality in a very beneficial way.

TRADITIONAL DREAM SYMBOLS

TO DREAM A FISH SWIMMETH ROUND IN THY CHAMBER
POT DOTH AUGUR VEXATION, BOTH FOR THE POWERFUL
MAN AND FOR HIM WHO AILETH.

Artemidorus Daldianus

E know that the personal unconscious acts as a receptacle for all the thoughts and impressions that have occupied your attention during waking hours, and quite often of things which may have escaped your attention, too. Anything that your waking mind has found troublesome is, in effect, mulled over subconsciously, clothed in a fresh guise, and re-presented to your conscious mind in a form which you may find more acceptable. Even if you fail to understand the symbolism, it is best to accept your dream with an open mind. It would be good to become able to assimilate everything as it comes, to understand everything we need to know, to cope with anything that may happen. The dreaming process initiated by the unconscious mind is working towards a whole and wholly human state, in which nothing need ever again be hidden from the waking mind, in which no impression need influence the psyche unfavourably.

Everything that happens in your dream is a symbol, and those which feature in personal dreams, on a personal level, will be personal symbols. They may not have the same meaning for anyone else. To dream of a black cat, for instance, may be a symbol of good luck to you; to someone else it may equally well be a symbol of bad luck; to one it may be a symbol of warmth and friendliness; to another, it may symbolize uncaring aloofness. In some countries where they eat cats, it may even be the symbol of a good meal!

But when they occur in dreams which have emerged into your awareness from that mysterious territory, the collective unconscious – from the great dreaming store which is common to all humankind – the symbols, although they too may represent something personal to yourself, may well be shared to some extent. Nobody can really fathom the depths of this great ocean of shared experience, which has been building up since our ancestors evolved from the beasts. Some of the shared symbols of our dreams may have originated even before that long-drawn-out process was complete, and may feature in the awareness of animals too: symbols relating to the basics of a natural life; sunrise and sunset; moonlight; heat and cold; the search for food; the threat of capture by enemies.

Some of the most frequently occurring dream symbols, that may be modified or disguised from case to case, but are more or less common to everyone, are listed here.

ABYSS

This primeval pit can take many forms: dreams of great heights, great depths, and the sensation of falling, are closely allied. It can appear disguised as a coalmine, a quarry, a hole in the road or backyard, an earth-closet, a deep pond, a whirlpool, the edge of a cliff; anything that has a similar shape, or a similar inert capacity to swallow up anyone unfortunate enough to drop inside. We have seen in Chapter 3 how it can represent the most basic of world images – the Creation, the fall from grace, the very fact of living on a material earth rather than sharing the world of immateriality with the angels. In these broad terms it can imply over-concern with materialistic interests, and a warning that the dreamer has been ignoring higher principles in favour of financial gain or social prestige.

In more specific terms, the symbol of the abyss represents the personal unconscious. It may be a general reminder of the constant cycling process that takes place continuously within the psyche. An abyss dream can warn against negative thinking, against neglecting to deal with matters which are your responsibility. It could be a stern warning against pushing personal problems on to others, when you should be dealing with them yourself during waking hours.

On a still more practical level, the abyss can represent fear of loss and a sense of danger, fear of losing your position at work or in society, or of losing your way professionally; something that you find worrying yet difficult to pinpoint. It can warn against giving way to impulses that you really consider undesirable, breaching your usual code of conduct. As the psychic container, the *yin*, it can symbolize femininity, and for a man it can highlight fears of sexual inadequacy. To dream of an abyss-like situation demands urgent attention to the circumstances of your daily life: a warning best not ignored.

See also Cave, Falling, Tunnel.

ACCIDENT

Nowadays, most dreams of accidents involve driving, or finding your car damaged. To dream you actually crash into another car, or seem to have been in grave danger of doing so when you wake, involves the use of symbols at a very basic level. Cars, mechanical travel, metal objects in general, all these are symbols of materiality, and when they are functioning well, they represent your own normal progress through life. But when accidents happen, or there is a risk of an accident, the implication is that either you or those close to you are in danger of material loss, of coming up against financial or legal problems.

To dream that someone else has damaged your car implies that another person is the one in trouble, but it involves a material situation which you yourself have built up. For instance, suppose you have retired and your son or daughter has taken over your business. To dream of finding your car smashed suggests that they seem to be mishandling the business which you have worked so hard to build up. To dream that you are driving when an accident involving another vehicle happens or is imminent, or there is a near-accident, perhaps involving a train at a level-crossing (a common dream situation), implies that your affairs are running up against unavoidable difficulties. The key factor, then, is your journey through life being impeded by material difficulties.

See also Driving.

ACTING

A dream involving anonymous actors performing may imply that others with whom you are associated are unreliable or insincere. If you are the one doing the acting, it is likely that you are the one who is not being altogether honest. But it commonly happens in dreams that the actors you see are recognizable characters from a favourite TV programme, or perhaps from some other medium if it has a definite meaning for you. In this case their presence in your dream underlines the feeling you have for them. If, for instance, you feel that a certain soap opera is typical of normal, everyday life, and if your dream features characters from that series, they are setting the scene for you as a normal, everyday situation. But if you feel the show represents a spiteful or deceitful attitude, for instance, then that kind of behaviour will be the context of your dream. Always remember your own feelings with regard to these dream figures: they will provide the clue.

ADVERSARY

This mysterious, threatening character is one of the archetypes of the collective unconscious, and can usually be identified as the personal shadow. The symbol represents any major factor that you have not been accepting in waking life, and allowed to build up in the subconscious mind until it has assumed menacing proportions. Any specific worry or temporary difficulty that has not been dealt with by your conscious mind may appear in dreams as an assailant rather than an adversary, which tends to have an ongoing nature. If you can recapture the essence of your dream (refer back to Chapter 5), try to face up to the image and identify it. Though menacing, it cannot really harm you – it is already a part of you. If you are a religious person, an image of the devil as an adversary may represent everything within your own character that you consider belongs to his department: everything that is undesirable. An aggressive or threatening figure, person or animal may carry some kind of identifying feature that will enable you to place it in terms of your work, or recreation, or family life. If you can isolate and name the fear, you will be better placed to handle it.

See also Assailant, Demon, Tunnel.

ALTAR

The centre of worship within your feelings, and the place that you would not want to see defiled with anything you normally dissociate from that feeling of devotion. Different people have differing principles, and are devoted to different things. At the heart of your feelings, symbolically, is the table of the altar, the *sanctum sanctorum*. It may be associated with the feelings you have towards another person, and is very often connected with a sexual relationship. Perhaps you feel that your relationship is not generally acceptable for one reason or another, and you would like to make it so. If you remember placing something on the altar in your dream, take careful note of it, and think round it. Remember also if anything was already on the altar. To summarize, the symbol represents either a principle which you already consider to be beyond reproach, or a circumstance that you would dearly like to make respectable, and free from guilt.

See also Church.

ANGEL

The world mandala in Chapter 3 hints at how angels may be regarded in relation to our everyday world. Within the psyche, they are the antithesis of the aggressive 'plant nature', and the competitive, amoral 'animal nature' in ourselves. As dream symbols, their presence balances the world of nature. Precisely what an angel means for you will depend almost entirely on your own experience of life, your own ideas of what constitutes 'an angel', and what you suppose the function of an angel to be. In most cultures they are thought of as messengers of God, and made of light. When their image is drawn from the collective unconscious, they are able to represent whatever the will of God is perceived to be by the individual, in any given set of circumstances.

Much depends upon what an angel means to you personally. In the West, it is usual to think of angels as gentle beings who might be relied upon to give a helping hand when it is most needed: loving, forgiving creatures, sexless and non-judgemental. But in some countries of the East, angels are thought of in an unsentimental way as divine administrators, doling out judgement, punishment or reward as it is deserved. There, they may be depicted as fierce, masculine creatures wielding a sword or battleaxe. In this case a dream angel may bear a message that the dreamer does not want to listen to in waking life. Suppose a dream angel appears in typical Western form: winged, robed, golden-haired perhaps, filled with love; this will be the message it carries – reassurance, condolence, possibly gentle reproof. Mystics say that angels, being made of light, can assume whatever form and appearance they wish. Should a *real* angel appear before you in your dawn dream, you should be in no doubt about the message: it will be for you alone.

ANGER

Anger can sometimes actually be seen in a dream, or in a waking vision, appearing like a dark cloud issuing from an angry character's mouth. It may sometimes be smelled as a rotten-plant smell. Dream anger is often expressed when someone, perhaps quite unconsciously, has pointed out some personal characteristic that may be acting as a barrier to smooth psychic functioning; they may have hinted at a flaw in the character of the person displaying the anger. Sometimes the emotion is transferred, so that the person who triggered it appears to be the angry one. Dream anger of this type means that the psyche acknowledges the fact that change is needed, but is unwilling to face up to it in waking life. Angry dreams always need personal interpretation by thinking round each element and theme, trying to identify the mental or emotional barriers which are sure to exist. 'Righteous indignation' is something of a conscious myth, and seldom if ever occurs in the dream world. Dream anger nearly always signifies that something is wrong; something that ought to be put right.

ANIMALS

Dreams in which the dreamer seems actually to be an animal may be reflections of the world dream (see Chapter 3), or may even hint at reincarnation, or 'dreaming another's dream' on an animal level (see Chapter 8). Somebody like a farmer, for instance, to whom animals are particularly familiar, may find that they are included in a dream merely to set the scene in familiar surroundings. But where this is obviously not the case, and animals have featured strongly in a personal dream, personal interpretation will be needed. Heavy, horned animals carry with them the idea of powerful masculinity best not disturbed, and as a simple warning, may suggest that the dreamer should take care in his or her daily life not to upset the kind of man who might fit this category. A wild forest animal, such as a startled deer among the trees, may be telling you that you have been evading social obligations, taking refuge instead in the 'forest of the mind'.

To dream of your own pet animals is often a fairly straightforward message regarding them. But many amazing examples of animal dreams have been recorded when the dreamer is setting out on a spiritual path (see Chapter 9). The shadow can take the form of a fierce animal, often a travesty or distortion of a domestic pet known to the dreamer. A frightening apparition, but a fairly common device which draws attention to the fact that this demonic creature in the dream represents something that is actually very close and familiar – a part of the dreamer's own subconscious, that has built itself up into this frightening form, and requires the dreamer's understanding.

See also Bull, Cow, Demon, Dog, Horse, Pig.

ASSAILANT

Broadly similar to the archetype of the adversary, the assailant represents matters which the dreamer has found challenging or disturbing, but has not been able to deal with during waking hours. Such things are invariably pushed into the inner feelings where they are liable to become absorbed by the shadow. A dream assailant tends to represent a one-off circumstance, something from outside oneself. A dream adversary tends to represent a permanent condition existing within the self. The actual nature or identity of your dream assailant tends to remain unknown, and it may be felt simply as an unseen, brooding presence. If you are able to re-enter your dream (see Chapter 5), you may be able to identify it and the dream itself may offer a solution. Even if you cannot do this, it may yield to your personal interpretation, by thinking round every aspect of the dream, by noting your emotions at every stage, and listing any associated themes that you find even vaguely upsetting.

See also Adversary.

BABY

The innocent child self is a major archetype of the collective unconscious. The symbol of a very young baby, however, is more likely to refer to some particular aspect of the self, to an unfamiliar inner dimension that has just been 'born', or come to realization. Otherwise, a baby may represent any new life, or new venture, new psychological direction, new career, new way of looking at yourself – anything that seems to have come newly to life.

See also Child.

BALL

Chapter 1 included the idea that the non-material self is in some ways like a ball; and the more one progresses towards wholeness, the more spherical will the self seem. But a ball, of course, is a common plaything for a child or a household pet, and its image can carry a hint of the carefree but not particularly helpful pursuits of others. This in turn can imply that the dreamer has felt left out of things, or isolated, physically or emotionally. Football, baseball, or other major games are so widely popular that they can carry dream significance with regard to relationships. A professional game can represent not recreation or strife, or competition, so much as the majority viewpoint. Everyone attending a match seems to be slanted in one specific direction, supporting their side. Songs and chants strengthen the feeling of 'all for one and one for all'. The ball sometimes seems to be the only odd one out. Dreams involving these things, therefore, can carry a powerful feeling that the dreamer is either firmly in or firmly out of step with the most widely held popular view, and is therefore in danger of ignoring the needs of some individual or minority group, or conversely of courting unpopularity by swimming against the tide of opinion.

BIRDS

Some people are frightened of birds; others love them and would like to spend most of their time thinking about them and watching them.

They are said to be direct descendants of the dinosaurs, so they can express the idea of a primeval life force. Birds, as members of the animal kingdom, tend to be competitive and parochial: they look after their own, putting family and group before the general welfare. Bird nature may be cold and selfish, but they are programmed to warn others by their cries when danger is about.

There is a host of meanings that have traditionally been associated with birds: the blue bird of happiness; the white dove of peace; the black raven of fate; the stork of childbirth; the owl of wisdom; the vulture of death; the freedom of the wild goose; the mindless repetition of the parrot; and the peacefully beautiful, such as a hummingbird, a sunbird, a kingfisher. A flock of birds can suggest migration, going to seek refuge in some faraway place, or arriving from afar. It might equally symbolize wasted efforts or natural catastrophe. Many a peasant farmer has watched helplessly as a flock of birds devours his precious crop, his past efforts, his family's welfare. Look at the biblical dream of the Pharaoh's master baker. His best efforts were brought to nothing and he was made to suffer the extreme penalty – all symbolized by birds eating the results of his work.

See also Animals.

BLOOD

For your physical body, blood is the essence of life; dreaming about blood has to carry an earthbound or materialistic message. Occasionally, whole nations seem fairly obsessed with the image of blood, their people seeing themselves as noble, long-suffering, and prepared for self-sacrifice. To this extent, the meaning of blood as a dream symbol will depend on your own cultural background. In dreams that reflect the world dream, it carries implications of aggression and selfish conflict. In the great majority of dreams of blood or blood-stained clothing, however, the implication is physical trauma, or possibly concern over illness involving the heart and circulatory system.

BOAT

A vessel sailing peacefully symbolizes safe passage over the depths of emotion, undisturbed by the more turbulent aspects of sexual attraction. The image of a stormy sea is closely connected with the boat symbol, and a storm almost invariably refers to stormy emotional scenes and wildly erratic relationships. As with any symbol of transport, it includes the basic idea of a journey, either in general terms, through life, or more specifically from one place to another. Large ocean-going liners featured in dreams may carry the simple practical message of overseas travel. For individuals who are connected with boats in their daily lives, the symbol may merely be setting the scene for their dream, placing it on a workaday basis.

BOOKS

Unless they are plainly antique and valuable in themselves, dream books tend to represent their own contents – and the idea of knowledge and information kept in store ready for use when required. They can symbolize virtue, wisdom, the knowledge of a learned person, or an academic institution of some sort. In spiritual dreams, an open book may reveal some information necessary for the dreamer's spiritual progress, in words or pictures. But usually in any dream there is the extra dimension of personal familiarity – what does the idea of books mean to the dreamer? To some, books in general may suggest education that is unavailable, something only the privileged few have access to. To others, books carry a more positive meaning: satisfaction, romance, reliability, sufficiency. A book is usually more than a simple scene-setter in a dream; it is a symbol that can be thought round, and interpreted according to the dreamer's personal experience and needs.

BRIDGE

A potent symbol, a dream bridge always represents the means to cross over or surmount some obstacle. A bridge over water calls for a personal interpretation of 'water', considering its clarity or muddiness, depth or shallowness, its sexual or emotional implications in the dreamer's waking life. Looking down from a bridge lays stress on whatever lies or flows beneath, and represents a convenient way of observing or appraising whatever may lie at the root of a problem: possibly something over which you feel aloof, or that you do not want to have direct contact with. The experience may carry a feeling of wistfulness, of wishing to become involved. Looking up at a bridge from below carries the opposite meaning: you, the dreamer, will be wondering how you can surmount your problems, wondering if you can climb up from the difficulties of your waking life. A bridge over another road or a railway can imply a feeling of superiority over the general run of humanity – or similarly a sense of longing that you could join in their activities. A bridge could feature in the dream of a 'fugitive' who feels isolated, and is looking for a way to rejoin the world at a more fulfilling level.

See also Path, Water.

BULL

A powerful animal, usually seemingly docile, but potentially violent and dangerous. On the level of the world dream, a bull epitomizes animal-based clannishness and difficulty of social access. A wholly male symbol, the dream bull often represents an actual person with overly masculine characteristics; a person who in normal times will 'live and let live', but who may prove a dangerous enemy if his interests are challenged, or if non-bullish ideas are introduced into his domain. As usual, interpretation must depend on the dreamer's own life experiences. A farmer, for instance, may have a special familiarity with bulls; a bull-fighter certainly will, and his imagery may be quite different from most.

See also Animals.

CALENDAR

Like the clock, a calendar symbolizes the passage of time, often expressing urgency and the need for action. It can be a reminder that time is limited, and there are things to be done. It may simply be reminding you of an important date or a forgotten anniversary. It may also symbolize the possibility of a change from the merely mundane level of dream experience, offering a hint of real spiritual contact. A calender, of course, can refer backwards as well as forwards: it may be drawing your attention to some forgotten event which has significance in your life today. When other dream images are involved too, they should be interpreted with dates and times in mind.

See also Clock.

CANDLE

Religions which make use of symbols often employ candle imagery, though candles, as a rule, play no part in the story of a religion, or the history of religious practices and beliefs. They are an extra that has been added chiefly for sentimental reasons. Those religious adherents who consider themselves to have direct contact with the divine seldom feel the need to make use of candle imagery. Others, less direct in their beliefs, adore candles and sometimes seem unable to get enough of them. On the face of it, a candle is something of a phallic symbol, and so implies fertility and rebirth. A religious dimension adds the fire of spirit: divine light that will point the way. In the West, a favourite theme of Christmas cards; in some cultures candles in containers are set to float on water – itself a symbol of emotional and sexual depths. Such customs go a long way towards explaining the candle as a dream symbol.

CARVINGS

Carvings or figurines in ivory or wood often feature as dream symbols of the collective unconscious, and usually carry the idea of ancient wisdom – or, equally, of old religious beliefs that may carry the outward appearance of wisdom, but lack spiritual reality. Often, a carving can be understood as a phallic symbol, and may refer specifically to a sexual relationship that the dreamer feels guilty about. There is usually a religious element to a carving which represents a human figure, and an animal carving too may represent something in the sense of 'the old religion'. It may be that the dreamer is being shown that the time has come to shed past unquestioned beliefs, and seek instead something with a more meaningful content. Identifiable carvings or statues which feature in a dream may, of course, have a special meaning to the dreamer. In this case significance may lie in the detail of the carving, or in the idea of carving or creating something tactile.

See also Statue.

CAVE

Connected with the abyss of materiality, as a cavity in the earth mother, this symbol can imply a place of refuge or concealment. For a man, it can also represent motherhood, and may point to the need for a young man to break away from his mother's dominating influence, to gain true independence. In the sense of an abyss, a cave may represent an unseen and unknown danger. In this case it will probably refer to contents of the personal unconscious, as part of the dreamer's shadow.

See also Abyss.

CHILD

In everyday dreams, of course, a child may represent a young family member without symbolic disguise. But in cryptic dreams the symbol of the innocent child usually represents, if not the whole self, then at least an aspect of one's personal contents, even though it will appear in the dream as a separate non-self individual. When spiritual progress is taking place, the child symbol may represent the dawning of a formerly hidden aspect of the self which must now be assimilated.

See also Baby.

CHURCH

When interpreting the symbol of a church, as with any symbol about which there is a hint of divinity, there are two distinct possibilities to bear in mind: it may represent the possibility of further spiritual progress, the path of submission to a higher will; or it may indicate an ancient and possibly redundant set of beliefs. In the first case, the dream church will be seen as growing and flourishing; in the second, as ruined, ivy-covered, abandoned and crumbling. Both are fairly common features in dreams, and both are 'good' symbols, in that they represent the dawning of new understanding in the dreamer's waking mind. Spires and steeples may carry the same implications, as may more abstract 'church' symbols, such as the sound of bells, singing or chanting. To dream one is entering a beautiful church and feel at peace implies one's arrival at a new level of understanding. As always, the full context of the dream, and the habitual lifestyle of the dreamer, should be considered and thought round when trying to analyse it. Unpleasant and disturbing dreams involving churches need urgent personal interpretation.

See also Altar.

CLIMBING

Climbing symbolizes valuable psychic progress if it seems to have successful results in the dream. If it results only in getting lost or in danger of falling, it is more likely to imply searching and doubt. It always requires interpretation with a spiritual journey in mind, and it usually calls for a change of attitude. A successful drive towards psychic wholeness involves a feeling of submission to the divine will. The personal ego may be following the mistaken belief that it can climb, alone and unaided, to the heights of 'objective daylight', but this is an illusion. The ego has no place in the spiritual heights, and the dreamer needs to be reminded of the world dream mandala. Dream-climbing within the material zone points to a mistaken attitude: the light towards which you climb is the misleading sunset light of Lucifer; there is no way through, and you are sure to fall back into the darkness. To be successful in spiritual terms, the dreamer needs to climb, not as an adult, but as a child – the child self, with a childlike attitude of acceptance. On a more mundane level of dreaming, involving work and the daily social round, to dream of climbing means that your drive towards material power and achievement may be successful, but it is not working towards wholeness of the self.

See also Mountain.

CLOCK

A symbolic timepiece points to triggers, opportunities, consequences and fate. The clock face itself is a mandala which can represent the dreamer's whole life. There comes a time in everybody's life when the alarm goes off and the fateful hour strikes, and the dreamer should be advised when such a moment is imminent. Two clocks together also have great significance in a dream: two lines of destiny have met in the space–time continuum – two people, perhaps – and this meeting point is the trigger for a new start, a new direction. The sundial is also a mandala of the self, and suggests a long and difficult life journey in the dreamer's past. With its gnomon and plinth, a sundial also carries a phallic significance, and suggests that a change in lifestyle is imminent.

See also Calendar, Mandala.

CLOTHES

A most important symbol. A person's clothes represent his or her sense of being, their persona, or social façade, their passionate content, the way they think of themselves, and the way others think of them. The symbol may refer to clothes worn by the dreamer, or by someone else featuring in the dream. Clothes, like an actor's costume, sum up the nature of the character. In dreams, important people, or non-personal principles and powers in the guise of people, normally wear impressive robes. Unknown quantities and suspicious circumstances may be represented by characters clad in shady, dark clothes. To dream that your own clothes are inadequate, or not smart enough, or that you can never find the right outfit to wear, implies that you do not feel able to fit into the social scene – it means you are lacking in confidence. Success in many fields depends upon confidence in one's own ability to fill the role; the dreamer whose clothes seem unsatisfactory should be helped to put on the new clothes of confidence in waking life. Others tend to take you at your own valuation, hence the symbol; you are judged by the appearance which you largely project for yourself. In more general terms, the dreaming self can be aware of clothes which sum up the waking situation for the dreamer: a sick person may dream of a figure dressed in red, the colour of blood; a widow may dream of a wedding in which the bride is dressed in black. A dream that involves unusual clothes always calls for personal interpretation.

See also Hat, Naked.

CLOUDS

By their nature, clouds are insubstantial, and usually high above the ground. As a dream symbol, they conceal whatever unknown situation is or may be above the normal state of the dreamer. Clouds differ from fog or mist which, as dream symbols, may conceal the future, and hide what is on or below the status of the dreamer. Storm clouds inevitably carry the idea of conflict, though it may not directly involve the dreamer. To dream that someone else passes through clouds in some way implies that they have progressed to a state that cannot yet be known by the dreamer.

See also Darkness, Fog.

COW

Domestic cattle have symbolic significance in many cultures. The symbol of the cow is liable to emerge from the collective unconscious as representative of motherhood in the sense of a sustaining mother earth – the fertility goddess who appears in many guises. By inference, cows can represent the regularity or reliability of nature, the natural bounty of the earth, good harvests and times of plenty. A herd of cows can also symbolize the nature of the figure who may be driving or leading them. This is likely to be one of the personal soul-children who will be described as a dream character in the final chapter.

See also Animals, Goddess.

CROSSROADS

We use this idea as a simile in everyday life, suggesting a point of decision, a time when our direction may change, a crucial stage when we are forced into making a decision about our future course. As a dream symbol, there is also an element of dubious behaviour or criminality about the crossroads for, in the past, in Europe at least, they were often chosen as places for meting out rough justice: criminals were hanged and buried there. Sacrifices too were often made there in ancient times, so as a crossing point of fate, their atmosphere was full of doubt or hidden danger. In some countries, crossroads have been thought of as meeting places for entertainment, and inns or eating-houses were often built there. So, besides the fateful choice that must be made, this symbol can carry the sense of a meeting between unrelated ideas.

CROWN

A symbol implying authority. The archetype of authority and wisdom may appear in your dream as a crowned man, and the mother goddess too may wear a version of this – more usually a tiara or headband. In dreams involving wakening of the soul (final chapter), a person known to the dreamer in real life may appear in the dream wearing a crown, indicating that he or she may be able to help in that important respect.

See also Clothes, Goddess, King.

CUP

A cup, or chalice, is a universal symbol of the collective unconscious, signifying preordained fate. In some cultures it may appear as a calabash, a drinking horn, or even a skull. To Christians, it tends to represent something unpleasant that must be done as a duty, and from which there is no escape. Jesus is said to have received the vision of a cup shortly before his arrest and crucifixion. In any culture it represents a fate, an unavoidable circumstance, that is about to descend on the dreamer. When the symbol takes the form of a bejewelled chalice of precious metal, it may well mean that something of great benefit to the dreamer is about to happen. It can also represent a feeling of divine approval of the dreamer's situation in waking life.

DANCE

There are many examples of ritual dance in the animal kingdom, mainly connected with the aim of mating. As dream images, some of these may become transferred to the personal awareness to signify courtship, or the sort of ritualistic behaviour many people use to conceal their true feelings. The 'lek' dance of the black grouse has been actually experienced in a dream, only to turn into a top-hat-and-tails courtship of the not-so-prim daughter of Victorian-minded parents. A more normal dance involving a group and modern dance-hall may best be interpreted according to the dreamer's own experience. Formation- or folk-dancing can also represent a mandala of the self.

See also Clothes, Mandala.

DARKNESS

As a dream symbol, darkness describes the unknown part of the self, the personal unconscious waiting to be explored through dreams. In fog or mist, your way forward is merely obscured or delayed. In darkness, rather than uncertainty, there is a sense of ignorance of, or alienation from, higher states of consciousness. Dreams of walking through a dark tunnel without apparent end may be experienced during the night, but dawn dreams of darkness are more likely to involve a glimpse of light as if at the end of a tunnel. Darkness is not necessarily a 'bad' symbol; rather a necessary and temporary stage along the route towards personal fulfilment.

See also Clouds, Fog, Tunnel.

DEATH

In dreams the image of death need not necessarily refer to death of the physical body. Factually predictive dreams of physical death, when they happen, and unless they can be taken as a warning to take evasive action, can only be accepted with equanimity as something over which we have no control. Paradoxically, however, all spiritual progress proceeds by way of psychic death, for death is the necessary precursor of rebirth. Eventually, we might even come to realize that the human soul, as the non-egoistic self, also has to face a process akin to death and rebirth in order to change for the better. As a dream symbol, therefore, death may imply a change from the old to the new, from the tired and outworn to the new and progressive.

See also Funeral, Tunnel.

DEMON

The archetype of the personal shadow: a representation of the contents of the personal unconscious, made up of the numerous ideas, impulses and characteristics which have been rejected or not recognized by the conscious mind. All the features, faults and failings of the subpersonality combine to create a symbolic figure which may assume many forms. It is liable to appear in dreams to haunt people who have begun to progress along the path to psychic wholeness, or to people who seek spiritual contact. It is a part of the psyche which seems *not to want* to come to awareness and, having taken on a will of its own, adopts a frightening guise in order to strengthen its own nature.

See also Adversary, Witch.

DESERT

To dream of travelling in the desert implies barrenness, either physically or spiritually. The symbol often reflects the dreamer's own feelings about the way their life seems to be going. A dream situation where no plants grow reflects a sense of being powerless, overwhelmed by events. Remember the world dream: you may obtain a seed which will germinate and grow in your dream desert, and transform it into an oasis. It is not impossible!

See also Path, Rocks, Valley.

DIRT

Your dreaming self is well aware of the contaminating properties of dirt; but dreams involving something particularly unclean need personal interpretation by the dreamer. Does the dirt come from someone else, or is it already a feature of the personal unconscious? The dream is certain to express this clearly, and there is a world of difference. It is natural for the personal shadow to contain all sorts of impurities which may not be acceptable to the dreamer's waking mind, and to become aware of this kind of dirt represents a cleansing process in itself. Efforts should be made to identify the true nature of this dream dirt, and possibly to transform it into something more positive.

See also Excrement, Weeding.

DOG

For thousands of years, dogs have appeared in dreams as symbols of the unconscious mind – or the underworld. They represent the 'human-animal' nature well, because they live with us, apparently sharing our sense of social status, fitting in with our way of life. Doggy instincts, or those of the wolf pack, often compare favourably with some of our own social customs. The personal shadow can take on the appearance of a dog in our dreams, letting its demonic nature be known only after it has been petted and accepted. When a clearing-out process has begun, re-creating the material that makes up the personal shadow, the dream symbol of a dog eating its own vomit is a warning against returning to former bad habits. In your own dream you will probably know if a dog is 'just a dog', or a part of yourself. Interpretation is bound to be a personal matter for the dreamer.

See also Animals, Demon.

DOOR

Passing through a dream door symbolizes experiencing or becoming aware of a different level of being, and it appears in example dreams elsewhere in the book. As a dream symbol, a door may open to reveal light, and is often associated with a near-death experience. The difference between a door and a gateway is that you can see through and round a dream gate; you know what lies beyond and merely wish to attain it. In the case of a door, whatever lies beyond is utterly unfamiliar and new. You do not as a rule know whether you want to go through it or not.

See also Gateway.

DRAGON

Interpretation of this symbol will depend almost entirely on the dreamer's personal and cultural background. What does a dragon mean to you? What kind of dragon is it? What feelings does it invoke in you?

If you have firm answers to any of these questions, you will probably be able to interpret its appearance in your dream. It may, however, be a denizen of the primeval swamp that is your own personal unconscious. Then again it may appear as the guardian of a mysterious cavern containing an unknown treasure – and this is also a part of yourself. Experience your own dragon and make a pet of it; you may then be shown the treasure.

See also Monster.

DRIVING

For a person who habitually drives a car, as a dream symbol driving represents one's personal progress through life. In dream-life, the car is seen merely as an extension of the legs, and is unlikely to represent a substantial journey. For people who do not drive, riding in a bus or train can also symbolize the dreamer's everyday progress through life. Driving a bus with passengers implies that the dreamer is, or feels, responsible for the welfare of others. A family man, for instance, might dream he is driving his family in a passenger vehicle. In such dreams, the circumstances encountered along the route will need personal interpretation.

See also Accident, Feet, Path, Rail journey.

DROWNING

In dreams, deep water symbolizes the depth of your emotions, including, very likely, your sexual feelings. If you are drowning in your own feelings, or are unable to cope with your own sexuality, your own powerful emotional attachments, you need to follow your dream through, if you can. Drown in the dream if you have to, or scramble ashore, but on waking try to identify the nature of the water, so that you are able to walk more safely round it in future. You might even be able to find a bridge enabling you to cross it in safety.

See also Water.

EXCREMENT

Not quite the same as dirt, human excrement inevitably symbolizes unwanted characteristics leaving the self. It clings where it touches, so try to dispose of it cleanly without getting fouled up.

See also Dirt.

FALLING

A very basic sensation which may feature in your dreams. Sometimes it happens to the sleeper without any apparent supporting dream. The image may correspond in some personal sense with the original plunge into materiality in the world dream. It always implies that a base, or attitude of mind which you thought was secure, is not as reliable as you hoped. It frequently happens that, as you feel the sensation of falling, you realize you are dreaming and wake yourself up. Determine to stay asleep if it happens to you again, and experience the conclusion of the fall. In the dreamworld, the consequence of falling is already part of you, part of the self, so you are not really escaping anything by waking up prematurely. Experience it again, identify its nature, and you may be able to deal with it in real life.

FEET

A potent symbol of the ability or inability to progress in spiritual terms. To dream that feet are missing or deformed may imply that your own wilful nature is impeding the long march towards psychic wholeness. To understand this symbol is to become aware that a journey is necessary. Become aware also that you must not impede the progress of others by trampling on them or kicking them. Live and let live! Wheels may carry much the same significance in a personal dream.

See also Path.

FLOWER

The symbol of a flower bears some relationship with the archetype of the persona – one's social façade. It can represent something that is being presented, the qualities that you are intended to see and experience regarding something or someone; also the way you want others to see you. The flower – especially a four- or five-petalled flower – can also symbolize the self, particularly when it is displayed full-face in the manner of a mandala. However, a flower that is set on a surface, like a water-lily floating on a pond, can symbolize the upper, conscious part of the self, above the dark contents of the unconscious mind. Strange or exotic flowers can represent some unusual encounter you have had, perhaps an unfamiliar religious attitude. Flowers in general can also represent the spiritual essence of the plant world, and so may reflect the world dream. Dreams of an afterlife frequently feature flowery meadows and gardens (see Chapter 9).

See also Clothes, Mandala.

FLYING

The inner feelings are your emotions below the horizon of consciousness – feelings that do not normally come to your waking awareness, though they are filled with all the matters that most concern you. When they do come to your awareness, usually in dreams, they do not feel themselves to be encumbered with the physical body, and there is nothing to stop them flying or floating freely. Aware of all your hidden potentials, they often draw the distinction in dreams between your outer and your inner emotions by personifying them. You may see yourself as two people, the one earthbound and heavy, perhaps with characteristics you do not care to call your own, the other able to float and fly, with ideal characteristics. This latter is the non-material part of you.

FOG

Doubt; not knowing what the future may bring; uncertainty of the best path to take. These negative feelings are symbolized by fog or mist. If we visit that great valley of materiality in our dreams, it will very likely be filled with fog, implying that spiritual light and wisdom are hidden from view. Experiencing fog in your dream does not imply that things will not improve for you; it simply means that a veil has been drawn over the future.

See also Clouds, Darkness.

FOREST

In dreams, a forest through which you are walking usually symbolizes the thoughts, the workings of your own brain. This is true particularly when your preconceptions are holding you back, or limiting your chances in some way. We tend to have fixed ideas which prevent us advancing in life. The minds of even great men and women are sometimes so powerful that they become scornful of matters which they consider illogical, religious or spiritual. Sometimes we need to relax our thoughts and seek higher things, and this is when the forest features most strongly in our dreams. In the great world dream the forest also represents the plant world, and is therefore associated with aggression and intolerance. As with most dream symbols, any practical interpretation should not be overlooked: if you have lived and worked in real-life forests, a dream forest may symbolize your own history and lifestyle.

FRUIT

The outcome of any enterprise or hopeful effort may be symbolized as fruit. The type of fruit will depend largely on your association of ideas: a tamarind, for instance, may symbolize good health in the East, but would be quite incomprehensible in the West. To Westerners, pears are frequently used by the dreaming self to represent bodily health. They can also represent one's own children. When the fruit is ripe and luscious, the omen is favourable; when it is shrivelled or rotten it implies disappointing results. Grapes and cherries in particular may indicate sexual attraction, and the phallic implication is fairly obvious when bananas and similarly-shaped fruit and vegetables are involved. Bear in mind too that these are plant symbols, and may imply selfish interests or hidden aggression.

FUGITIVE

The dream of the outsider who would dearly like to be admitted to a more comfortable situation in life. To dream that one is hiding, afraid of capture, or longing to rejoin a community is a powerful symbol expressing a burning desire to experience the life of the wakened soul. When the possibility of this event approaches, dreams often carry an impression of the fugitive watching and waiting, or gazing wistfully like a lonely child.

FUNERAL

Waking thoughts of death will often produce the dream symbol of a funeral, but it is not necessarily to be taken literally. It always implies the possible end of some circumstance. Old-fashioned dream books usually assert that a funeral portends happiness to come; the end of a bad period and the rebirth of a better one. Personal interpretation will usually decide if this is the case. When thoughts of death are on the mind, the details of a dream funeral can carry significance. It happens quite often that what appears to be an actual funeral turns out to be only a 'dress-rehearsal' of the ceremony, indicating imminent recovery from a life-threatening condition.

See also Death.

GATEWAY

Allied to the symbol of a forest, a gateway leading from the trees into the open symbolizes a way of attainment, of escaping from the restrictions of thought, and possible entry into a higher mode of understanding. A gateway expresses the need for a new intellectual approach in any field of experience. It may be significant if the dreamer actually passes through the dream gate, or merely looks through it, or is no more than aware of its presence nearby. A door has a similar significance, but is usually a more 'inward' symbol. Where the gate refers to a new way of thinking and receiving impressions, a door implies entry into a different dimension – often associated with an 'afterlife' experience.

See also Door, Forest.

GODDESS

The earth mother, or a goddess, is one of the archetypes of the collective unconscious, normally occupying for a woman the same position as the king, or hero figure, does for a man. The great earth mother may appear to either sex as a symbol expressing a first inkling of the reality of the world dream. On a more personal basis, the symbol represents a personification of female confidence and strength. It carries the implication of caring for others, sometimes to the extent of overruling the real-life independence of children and others. The symbol needs personal interpretation according to the context of the dream.

GOLD

As a symbol, gold has two different extremes of meaning. The common denominator is its great value. Gold can symbolize the material wealth of the earth which, in religious terms, is to be found within the satanic realm. It can also symbolize spiritual wealth. Golden garments equally may symbolize great authority and respect on earth – or the divine authority of angels, and the attainment of 'Buddha consciousness'. The dream image of gold, therefore, as old-fashioned dream books often assert, can suggest that undue attachment to material gain may result in long-term loss and disappointment; it may equally refer to the achievement of some sort of enlightenment.

See also Jewels, Pearl.

HAT

If someone has more than one line of interest – say he is both social worker and marine biologist – we might say: 'He's wearing his social worker's hat today!' The dream symbol is similar; it identifies the type of person wearing the hat, whether authoritative or disreputable, and what function they represent, also how they want you to see them. Archetypes of the unconscious mind are often to be identified by their hats. Where the dream subject is feminine and the hat, or lack of it, seems important, remember that in many cultures women are

97

considered wanton or immoral if they go hatless in public. It can therefore symbolize virtue and morality.

See also Clothes.

HERO

This archetype of the unconscious mind is related to the image of the wise man, and that of the king. The hero in dreams usually symbolizes part of the self that occupies the highest position in the personal mandala. It is the opposite of the personal shadow, and opposes it in dreams. It includes everything of yourself that you consider to be admirable, brave and reliable. Superman and Batman are cartoon projections of the symbolic hero.

See also King, Wise person.

HORSE

In dreams a horse often represents your own sexuality, or that of a husband or child. In the world mandala it occupies the competitive but moral animal sector: a white horse often symbolizes a person of whose sexuality the dreamer is nervous, but whom they nevertheless trust. A black horse represents an unknown quality of animal passion. The unicorn is a closely related symbol, and this may be seen as a horse that, besides sexuality, also bears something of a spiritual status. Both have a powerfully emotional inference.

See also Animals.

JEWELS

The symbol of a chest of jewels, or similar treasure of great value, tends to feature in dreams investigated by psychoanalysts, to be interpreted in various ways. Unlike gold, jewels almost inevitably symbolize good things which come by way of materialistic rather than spiritual pursuits. As a rule dreams in which they appear need to be analysed on a personal basis.

See also Gold, Pearl.

KING

A male archetype related to the hero and the wise man, the king symbolizes the part of the psyche that is seen as the seat of wisdom and accumulated knowledge. In a woman's dreams, a king-like figure may be the animus, or father figure. The king's exalted place is usually taken by the dream figure of a wise goddess or the earth mother.

See also Goddess, Hero, Wise person.

LOST

It is quite common to dream that you are lost. You may be walking in the dream along a familiar route, then suddenly lose your sense of direction, forget where you have to go or where you came from, and everything seems unfamiliar – or *almost* familiar. You may find yourself in a place well known to you as a child, and think about going home, only to realize that home is not there any more. Dreams involving dying or the premonition of death often include this aspect. The symbol draws our attention to the fact that there is more than one dimension to life, and that your spiritual side should be awake, and able to find the right direction. Even on the most mundane level, the symbol can imply that you have lost direction in your professional or family life; but the non-egoistic meaning is always inherent in the dream. The self has unlimited capacities for expansion, but this is not the department of the ego, which is limited to physical life on earth.

MANDALA

A symbol of the self. In dreams this can take many forms, besides a mere diagram on a piece of paper. It can be represented, for instance, by a folk-dance in which the participants form a square or a circle; by a city square with trees and people, perhaps seen from above; by an ancient stone circle; by a flower; by almost any symmetrical arrangement, in fact, usually with a clearly identifiable centre and four corners. Dream symbols such as this often call for sympathetic assistance in personal interpretation. When the self is seen in symbolic form, it implies a growing awareness in the dreamer of the possibility of seeking spiritual contact.

MONSTER

It sometimes happens that you deliberately avoid doing something which you would rather enjoy, but which you think you ought not to do; you may have an interest that you would rather no one knew about; something which you had thought belonged safely to your past may stir in you again. Any of these things may well be symbolized in your dreams as a monster, or some creature like a crocodile crawling out of a primeval swamp. It belongs to the topmost part of the shadow, a mobile part which can quite easily crawl upwards into your conscious life at any time. The best plan is to identify this monster, draw it from its swamp and look at it, appraise it and come to terms with it, and it may then no longer worry you.

See also Abyss, Adversary, Dragon.

MOUNTAIN

Any barrier, real or imaginary, physical or psychological, may appear symbolized in dreams as a mountain or mountain range, or a cliff-face which needs to be scaled. The same symbol may also represent not a barrier but new heights which the dreamer feels need to be conquered. Depending on one's own attitude and development, a mountain may represent at the one extreme the spiritual heights of sainthood or, at the other, the satanic heights of materiality. To dream of walking over a mountain or hill-top implies an awareness of hard, slow progress through life currently being experienced, with the promise of an improved – downhill – situation later on.

See also Climbing, Path.

NAKED

Inhibitions belong to the emotions, the normal outer feelings; the inner feelings are free from inhibition. Some people habitually see themselves as naked in their dreams and this circumstance, as far as other dream characters are concerned, seems perfectly natural. But sometimes it seems to be an issue in itself. Where clothes symbolize the trappings of the psyche, the passions, the social disguises, the emotional veneer we tend to wear in company, nakedness symbolizes the absence of these features. Thus to dream that you are naked and unashamed in company means that, in the dream, you are presenting yourself as you really are, without pretence. But if your sensations in the dream are unpleasant, and you feel the need to hide, it implies that you have been forced by circumstances to drop your disguise; possibly an unfortunate situation that you have arrived at by acting against your own better judgement.

See also Clothes.

PATH

One of the most ancient of dream symbols: your own path through life. Driving your car, or riding your bike, may have the same meaning. How the symbol is best interpreted depends on what is encountered along the way, and on the difficulty or ease of travel in the dream. These factors will reflect your own ability to cope with the problems you meet from day to day.

See also Driving, Mountain, Rail journey.

PEARL

A pearl of great price symbolizes a non-material treasure. Pearls in nature are produced by oysters under the sea; in symbolic terms, deeply

hidden within the emotions, at the very bottom of the personal mandala, actually within the concealing armour of an ancient, primitive
life-form, in the darkest part of the self: the personal shadow. When
the oyster yields up its treasure, the dreamer will have found a means
of penetrating the hidden emotions, re-creating those dark contents to
make the self complete and whole. The spherical shape of a pearl, too,
carries the significance of evolution within the world dream.

See also Gold, Jewels.

PIG

A symbol of highly variable significance, for pigs occupy a prominent
place in the feelings of most people of the world. As a dream symbol,
the impact will be powerful, but it will depend entirely on the
dreamer's own cultural background. The crux of the matter is, a pig
is an intelligent creature with many similarities to the human animal.
A wild boar occupies a rather different category, and will represent
untamed animal passions, but a domestic pig will represent, to one, a
familiar and valuable source of food; to another, because of religious
proscription, it will seem the epitome of evil. Notoriously greedy, it
will be seen by some as a living dustbin. Pink and naked, pigs and
piglets as dream symbols can represent sexual peccadillos. An interesting symbol, but one which calls for careful and tactful interpretation.

See also Animals.

POLICE

When someone has started along the 'path of purification', through
psychological individuation or spiritual contact, the dream symbol of a
policeman often appears: a warning or safeguard against temptation
when mistakes may be repeated. To dream of carrying a friendly
policeman in your car means that you have made or are about to make
a morally correct decision.

RAIL JOURNEY

Whereas a car journey, nowadays, signifies one's passage through life,
the car representing merely an extension of the legs, a train journey
usually symbolizes a more definite movement from one place to
another, a transition from one lifestyle to another. The meaning of this
symbol does vary according to the dreamer's own experience of train
journeys. People who normally commute daily by train may give this
symbol an entirely different meaning.

RIVER

The Jordan river for centuries has represented the barrier between life and death in the Christian world, and any river appearing as a dream symbol can have a similar meaning for people of any other religion or none. More usually, however, a river signifies the flow of emotions; more specifically, the flow of sexual desires. Crossing a river, or looking at one with a view to crossing it, is a common dream experience for people who have consciously begun to travel along the path towards psychological individuation, or spiritual purification; that is, when the cycling process of their own personal self, expressed by the mandala, is in positive motion and working towards wholeness.

See also Death, Water.

ROCKS

A rocky place is typical of dream symbols expressing the life-force of materiality. The implication is spiritual barrenness. To be travelling through a rocky place implies that this is a temporary phase soon to be surmounted.

See also Climbing, Desert, Valley.

SNOW AND ICE

Walking through snow and ice implies passing through a wintry, difficult time, but one that will, by its nature, shortly pass into spring. Steady progress through snow and frost and ice is usually a good omen of progress in the right direction. It advises patience on the part of the dreamer, and perseverance at whatever he or she is finding wearisome in waking life. As with most symbols, the meaning will be modified by the dreamer's personal experiences and expectations, but temporary hardship is the common factor.

STATUE

A human likeness which is also an object of materiality, the symbol of a statue may carry much the same meaning as a solitary standing stone – the personal self, and the urgent need for a change within the psychic centre of gravity. A statue may also represent an archetype which seems to have become petrified or frozen in time through disuse; a human function that has long been overlooked. The symbol may carry a phallic significance, particularly when it seems small enough to be held in the hand. Personal interpretation is required within the context of the dream.

See also Carvings.

STONE CIRCLE

An ancient mandala symbol of the self in its relation to the world and the solar system. It can also signify the family circle, particularly when the family is perceived as unyielding and morally stringent. There is frequently a sense of having to pass through the stones, as through a gateway, to a new understanding or level of being. The implication is one of ancient wisdom, waiting to be discovered. Whether the dream circle is large and well organized, such as Stonehenge, or merely a rough and overgrown circle of stones among the hills will depend largely on the dreamer's own background and experience. The symbol is less complete when it features only one isolated standing stone. But it is still a powerful symbol of the self, and usually accompanies the waking realization that a new religious outlook is required by the dreamer.

See also Mandala.

SUN

Probably the most ancient and abiding symbol of life and spirituality. A rising sun signifies the rebirth of the psyche to a new understanding or opportunity. The sun shines on all aspects of life unless they are hidden from view, so sunshine can symbolize openness in behaviour and relationships, depending on the context of the dream. A setting sun marks the passing of an old era; it implies a sense of peace with longing, and may symbolize the desire to seek higher principles of life. In the world mandala the setting sun sinks into materiality before re-emergence, and the symbol also calls for patience and acceptance on the part of the dreamer.

THORNS

Representing perceived danger and difficulties, they can also symbolize persecution and unfair discrimination as sensed by the dreamer.

TIDAL WAVE

A specialized aspect of water as a dream symbol. Waves of emotion, or a great wave of sexual desire – these are the implications to be read into it. You, as the dreamer, should recall what effect the wave had on the surroundings, on other people in the dream, on everything that was apparently non-self, and compare this with the effect that it had on you. If the wave swamps you and sweeps you away, it is time for serious reappraisal of your lifestyle. If you were not personally swamped by the wave, the implication is that, though the way ahead may be tricky, you will surmount your difficulties safely.

See also Water.

TUNNEL

As a symbol, this is related to the abyss and the cave. Travelling through a tunnel commonly features in dreams of death, indicating a period of uncertainty in the passage between this world and the next. In Buddhist descriptions of this symbol, several colours may appear, shining at various points along the tunnel, each representing a possible 'place of rebirth' within sectors of the world mandala. A tunnel inevitably symbolizes a state of uncertainty and period of transition. When there is a glimmer of white light at the end of a dream tunnel, the implication is that the dreamer's situation will greatly improve before long. As a waking exercise, after experiencing this dream, try transposing the image of a tunnel on to the world mandala, and try to visualize in which direction you are travelling.

See also Abyss, Cave, Darkness, Death, Valley.

VALLEY

A common symbol of materiality, particularly if it is shrouded in fog or mist. Related to the symbol of the tunnel, it portrays a lack of spiritual influence in your life, and signals a need to follow your own dreams through territory that is less oppressive. Start looking for a way out of that desolate, symbolic valley!

See also Desert, Fog, Rocks, Tunnel.

WATER

There are many forms which the water symbol can take: the sea, waves, rivers, streams, lakes, ponds, wells, or as drinking water in a cup, or the hollow of the hand. Personal interpretation of the whole dream should never be neglected, even if the meaning of the symbol itself may seem obvious. The feelings, the emotions, are symbolized in dreams by water; it follows that the clarity or murkiness of dream water is significant. Psychological lumber that has not yet been dealt with in the personal unconscious will darken and discolour the water with mud. Clear water with coral, shells and clean pebbles signifies crystal-clear emotions, with not too many psychological blocks holding the self back from its steady progress towards wholeness. Murky water suggests that attention should be given to your own inner condition, and recording and analysing your dreams is a good start. The first step towards solving a problem often amounts to acknowledging that the problem exists.

In the symbolism of the East, a hermit living on the banks of a mighty river is one who practises celibacy; in his case, the river represents his sexual desires. In Western symbolism, a river can represent death, and crossing it means leaving life's passions behind. To experience difficulties in crossing a river or stream in your dream may mean that you are reluctant to abandon old sexual habits which you would be better off without. It may also mean that you are unwilling to experience your own emotions to the full, and tend to switch off when emotive subjects are raised.

A restricted or contained area of water is likely to symbolize the inner self. A flower such as a water-lily floating on the lake can be pointing out that the dreamer is placing too much reliance on his or her intellect, or practising emotional self-control, while neglecting the deep water of the personal unconscious beneath the flower. The personal shadow which lurks in the depths of the lake may be growing in strength. The subconscious mind can also be symbolized by a well, which carries a symbolic representation of a store of wisdom waiting to be drawn. To drink water implies that the dreamer is taking in whatever is being symbolized by the water; overcoming personal problems can be represented in this way. The collective unconscious can be symbolized by a vast sea, and swimming in or tasting the water implies familiarity with its contents – perhaps even to the extent of drinking the entire sea! But a gentle drink of water held in the palm of the hand may symbolize a taste of wisdom, while appreciating the need to follow good advice.

See also Boat, Drowning, River, Tidal wave.

WEEDING

When the dreamer is conscious of the need to 'purify out' various faults and features that have become deeply ingrained, and is finding it far from easy, weeding a flowerbed will often feature as a dream symbol. Long underground roots, and mat-forming weeds invading other plants, portray the undesirable characteristics that may be affecting the dreamer's life, and are themselves very extensively, very deeply rooted in the inner feelings. Patience and perseverance are called for.

See also Dirt, Excrement.

WISE PERSON

An archetype of the unconscious mind, the wise person is a part of the self that tends to be called upon when carefully thought out decisions are needed. In dreams it may appear as a teacher, a doctor, the dreamer's father, or other authoritative figure, ready to give advice. It is associated with the images of the king, the goddess and the hero.

See also Hero, King.

WITCH

An archetype of the unconscious mind which corresponds to the personal shadow, and is a feature of the female self. The witch comprises all those hidden characteristics of which the individual is ashamed, or has denied, or would rather not consider as her own. These have continued to exist on a subconscious level until they form a powerful presence – the female equivalent of the evil Mr Hyde – which can make itself known when its owner 'loses control'. Some people, of course, understand 'witch' rather in the sense of 'goddess', as legitimately expressing their sense of religion and their awareness of the possibility of inner development. Any apparent contradiction mainly reflects word usage rather than dream imagery.

See also Adversary, Demon.

SEVEN

DREAMS OF THE FUTURE

AND BEING WARNED IN A DREAM THAT THEY SHOULD NOT
RETURN TO HEROD, THEY RETURNED TO THEIR OWN
COUNTRY BY A DIFFERENT ROUTE.

Matthew: 2, xii

TO most people, a dream of the future implies a 'warning dream'. But simply perceiving something of the future by way of dreams is not a particularly unusual event. Straightforward dreams of what is to be, usually relate to two or so days ahead. We could say that the inner self possesses this awareness within itself; it is able to see ahead of the physical body, both in time and space, and in a material, practical sense. The more aware we become of our own inner self, the closer this awareness of the future comes to our surface minds. In some cases it can even become part of the normal waking awareness, and when this happens, we might say that such a person has become 'psychic'.

Dreaming dreams of the future is not really an 'ability', and cannot realistically be considered a 'neglected function' of the physical brain. Scientific attempts to pinpoint such things experimentally soon become bogged down. Prediction of this sort is not itself predictable, and cannot be stage-managed. The experience is always more impressive than the theory, and carries its own conviction. The difficulty we have in understanding non-material issues arises because science, with its practical explanations and its proofs, can operate only within the sphere of materiality. To a logician, anything that belongs outside this sphere has the misleading appearance of a free ball that anyone can kick about at will.

Dreaming cannot be a 'predictive art', practised intentionally. Becoming aware of the future through dreams cannot be other than involuntary, and the will cannot play any part in them. Such dreams have to be spontaneous. You may, perhaps, wish fervently to know about something in the future, whether or not such and such will happen, whether you will succeed or fail; but dreams which seem to give you the information you want are always suspect, for they may be simply the products of your own wishful imagination. Like the lucid dreams and the wish-fulfilment dreams described in Chapter 5, your own ego may force its attentions on to the inner feelings, and try to 'swing' the dream, hoping to influence results. Fervour, anxiety or intense desire always render predictive dreams dubious, because they do involve the ego: the quiet voice of wisdom is easily overruled.

WHAT'S GOING TO WIN THE BIG RACE?

If we could dream reliably of what is to happen, simply because we would like to know, bookies would quickly go out of business. But involuntary dreams, even of this type, are quite well known. Very often, however, it seems as if our own inner feelings are having a joke at the expense of our conscious minds, providing cryptic clues which can only be untangled when it is too late to profit from them. My mother has often retold the story of this dream which she had when I was a little boy, shortly before World War 2:

> ℭ I dreamed that I and several other people were standing on the floating dock at the Liverpool landing stage, when suddenly it started wobbling, and the water of the River Mersey came splashing over the side of the dock. One of the harbour officials said, 'Don't worry, it's only the battleship!' 'Oooh!' everyone said. 'The battleship!' We watched as the grey ship sailed down the middle of the river, which was very wide at that point.

About ten o'clock the following morning my father made up his mind to take mother to Liverpool, to see the Grand National at Aintree. They enjoyed the first two races without picking a winner; then came the big race. They chose a fairly short-priced horse, which came in fourth, and they missed the winner – a rank outsider, a grey horse called Battleship. It was only on the way back home that she remembered her dream.

A PERSONAL CRISIS

A coincidence, you say? It could well be: that is exactly the trouble with the more everyday type of dreams which seem to relate to the future. To anyone hearing about such a dream, it could very well be no more than 'just coincidence', especially if the dreamer did not understand the dream well enough at the time, or take heed of it in time to make use of it. Comparatively minor dreams of the future, or warning dreams, furthermore, are often of so personal a nature that they could not really make sense to anyone except the dreamer. To an outsider, they could 'mean anything'! But the dreamer *knows* that it is indeed a true dream, and that the message is a very real but personal one, for them alone.

Occasionally we hear of tragic personal events foretold in dreams, but for obvious reasons they are not widely spoken of, though they may well modify a survivor's general attitude towards life and death. There is, for instance, the case of a little girl who told her parents about a dream in which she was swimming underwater, shortly before she tragically drowned. If there is a deep purpose to such dreams, we can only guess what it is.

Often, without the element of tragedy, the event foretold by a dream will have significance only to the dreamer or to the immediate family circle, and the telling of it will not 'travel well'. The details in some cases, if the people concerned were identified, could prove embarrassing or downright hurtful. The following is one strictly anonymous example of a domestic tiff foretold by a dream, an interesting mixture of cryptic dream-clue and literal fact:

In the dream I was standing on a railway station platform as a train came in, and passengers were bustling about. Then a voice said: 'Look, there's Trevor Huddleston!' I looked, and sure enough there was the tall figure of Bishop Huddleston, just off the train with his luggage. He was carrying an African child cradled in his arms. Then the dream changed, and I was in some rooms. Suddenly a rhino came charging in, knocking my things flying and trampling on everything as I dodged out of the way.

Bishop Trevor Huddleston, of course, was a staunch opponent of racism, and wrote the anti-apartheid book *Naught for Your Comfort*. I thought it was rather appropriate in my dream that he was carrying an African child. The following Sunday, a couple of days later, I was reading the paper when I came across a short paragraph: 'Bishop

Huddleston has arrived back in England from Africa, to take up his new position as . . .' I thought, 'Ha! Look out for the rhino!' Almost immediately my partner rushed into the room in a furious temper. She rampaged through my things, hurling my books on the floor and down the stairs, then deliberately trampled on them. I *still* have no idea what had upset her (it might have been 'PMT'), but she *did* apologize later.

PHARAOH'S DREAM

This chapter opened with a quote from the Bible – a brief, matter-of-fact mention of the warning dream of, presumably, all three Wise Men. Probably the best-known example of a warning dream of future events is the biblical Pharaoh's dream of cows coming up out of the river, predicting a devastating long-term drought for Egypt. It was certainly an unusually long-term prediction, if the story is true, relating to fourteen years ahead: seven years of plenty, to be followed by seven years of drought. It is a dream that could be analysed quite simply, following the method outlined in Chapter 2. If such a dream should crop up again, remember that you don't have to be a Joseph (of the many-coloured coat) to interpret it. We can all do as well quite easily. The dream, related in modern language, was as follows:

> I was standing in a meadow on the banks of the Nile, and some cows came up out of the river and began to graze. There were seven cows; the number was definite and seemed very important. They were fat, sleek and very healthy-looking, and they grazed contentedly in the meadow. Then seven more cows came up out of the river, but this time they were painfully thin, as though starving to death. Instead of eating the grass they ate up the fat cows, swallowing them whole. And when they had finished eating them, they still looked as thin and starved as before.
>
> Then I woke up. But while I was puzzling about it, I went to sleep again, and this time I dreamed of stalks of wheat. The first stalk had seven ears of wheat, and they were full of fat seeds and healthy. Then another stalk grew up, and this too had seven ears of wheat on it, but they were in very poor condition, thin and withered and quite useless. The poor-quality ears of wheat seemed to eat up the good ones, so that we were left with just the shrivelled, useless ears of wheat. Then I woke up again.

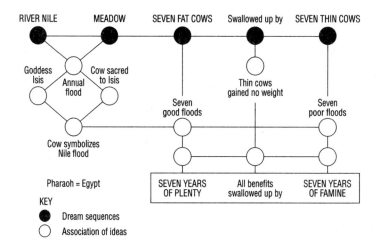

The Pharaoh was thought of as the living incarnation of Egypt, so his dream was, in effect, a collective dream for the whole country. These are the thoughts that might have come to Joseph, when asked to interpret the dream: the Nile was the great river upon which the whole life of Egypt depended; its annual floods were essential for the irrigation of harvests and grazing land. Joseph would have reasoned too that, in the Egyptian pantheon, Isis was goddess of the Nile, and annual floods were thought to be sent by her. The cow was considered sacred to Isis, and she herself was often depicted as having a horned head. The dream meadow by the Nile was, of course, the ground which the Nile could make rich, or barren. The condition of the cows coming up from the river represented the quality of the annual flood, each cow representing the good or bad fortune of any particular year.

As though to 'make assurance doubly sure', the ears of wheat in the second part of the dream symbolized the corn harvest suffering the same fate as the rearing of cattle. On its own, perhaps, the idea of an ear of corn devouring another ear of corn would seem fairly incomprehensible. But following immediately after the dream of cows, it was made abundantly clear: seven years good; seven years bad. This was to apply to the entire spectrum of agriculture alongside the Nile, cattle and wheat, meat and bread. Joseph's advice to the Pharaoh was to store all the surplus stock harvested during the fat years – but this was purely political, and had no place in the dream itself.

111

ONCE-ONLY WARNINGS

Major warning dreams of events on a national, or even a worldwide catastrophic scale may well derive from a wholly impersonal spiritual source, and perhaps the Pharaoh's dream falls into this category. The world of spirit is not penetrable by human minds, however clever, and such dreams will probably remain a mystery. 'Ordinary' dreams of forthcoming disasters, however, have to stem from the inner feelings of the personal inner self. Many people who experience persistently recurring dreams relate them to future events; but, unless unusually detailed, such dreams are usually far too vague of content, and the connection with anything happening in real life is too tenuous to be plausible. If you dream of falling often enough, for instance, and for a long enough time, the dream is likely to come true one day when you actually trip over the cat, or fall off the stepladder.

In my experience, however, the inner self, while concerned about the course of your life on earth, does not seem at all worried even by the forthcoming death of the physical body. Perhaps this is why 'disaster dreams' often seem inappropriately casual, one-off affairs. The chief characteristic of recurrent dreams, again in my experience, is that they are concerned with relaying something that should be known and put right about the dreamer's personal unconscious, a persistent inner condition, a refusal to face facts, or a loss of direction in life. To the dreamer, understandably, there will probably seem no doubt about it: when a comparable event occurs in real life, the recurring dream will seem to have proved itself. The following is a rather typical example:

> ℂ I dreamed that I was on a railway line in thick fog. Ahead of me was what appeared to be a tunnel, or a bridge, which had blood dripping down from it. This dream recurred for a whole year, until the event.
>
> I and my young niece were travelling on the Arlburg express, having been visiting relations in Austria. In the early hours of the morning our train crashed into another stationary train – the Frankfurt to Paris express. I climbed out on to the track after making sure my niece was all right. It was very foggy. There was wreckage, luggage and blood everywhere. What I had thought was a tunnel or a bridge in the dream was a coach piled on top of another. I learned later that twenty people had been killed, and forty injured. I never had the dream again.

I have no reason to doubt the dreamer's account, or his sincerity. But this time I must join the sceptics in the 'just a coincidence' brigade.

Convincing dreams that warn of future events seldom occur earlier than two days beforehand. Nevertheless it is interesting that they seldom seem to call for evasive action; they are more likely merely to be informative. The inner consciousness, probably of us all, is largely aware of future events as they affect ourselves and those close to us, and often seems more concerned with setting right small matters of conscience even than with the approaching death of the dreamer. Dreams that *do* call for evasive action on the part of the dreamer sometimes use devious means to bring it about.

WHITE LIES

When you become familiar with the language of dreams, you may discover that the message which you have received is untrue – but that it has apparently been planned that way for a very good reason. It is a surprisingly common ploy of the inner self to use a 'white lie' to persuade you to heed the real message. The following is an example of a 'white lie dream':

€ The night before I was due to travel by coach to see my sister in Edinburgh, I dreamed I was reading some newspaper headlines: 'Motorway Carnage', with pictures of vehicles upside down and piled on top of one another. Then it seemed to turn into a TV report, showing injured people being helped away from the road and through some fields.

I woke with a feeling of panic, and promptly changed my plans for the day, and put off the visit. Later in the day I rang my sister's house to make an excuse for not coming, but I had difficulty in getting through. It turned out that she'd had a house fire that morning, an hour or two after my coach was due to leave, causing extensive damage to the building and its contents. The firemen and police were in charge when I rang. They said she was unhurt and arranging to stay at a nearby hotel, and passed on my message. She certainly could not have coped with me as a visitor as well as all that hassle! Whether there actually was a motorway smash, I don't know. And I'm not sure either if the dream was truly a warning dream or not. But whether it was meant that way or if it was no more than nonsense, it certainly had the effect of preventing a great deal of unnecessary inconvenience.

It makes sense. Supposing the dreamer had dreamed of the actual event – a house fire at her sister's. She would have rung up straight away in the morning, and of course there would have been no fire − not yet. The call, and the dream, would probably not have helped to prevent one. The dream would certainly have 'proved itself' when the fire actually occurred − but this is not the point of dreams. The inner self has nothing to prove, and has absolutely no desire either to make a name for itself as a prophet, or to trivialize itself as a mere fortune teller. As effectively as possible, the dream said: 'Don't go!' and it worked.

SEEING AS IN A DREAM

People who have experienced soul-awakening (see Chapter 9) sometimes have what might be termed 'waking dreams' of future events. The inner feelings, in touch at last with everyday consciousness, show them what is to be. The closer the contact between inner and outer awareness, the more vivid, and by that fact the more 'unremarkable', will such experiences seem.

Waking perceptions of the future can be quite down-to-earth and everyday. They are often *almost* simultaneous, giving time enough for evasive action, if required. A car driver might 'see' a hedgehog cross the road, preparing him to avoid the real-life hedgehog when it actually appears a few seconds later; or he might 'see' a lorry approaching at dangerous speed along a narrow country lane − while still out of sight. Experiences like this are not actual dreams, of course: they are of the same stuff. They are the simple observations of that part of the self that is normally unconscious. Such perceptions may quite frequently be connected with the grim but inevitable prospect of death, because death is a major event, though it holds no fears for the inner consciousness. The example that follows is *not* a dream, though it could well have been. It was an incident arranged by the inner self − an encounter between two souls relaying a pictorial message:

> I was doing some work in a local churchyard, and stopped to pass the time of day with the verger. He was standing rather awkwardly, strad-dling a piece of ground which I guessed was probably a vacant grave-plot he had to locate. As we chatted I felt very sympathetic because, to me, his face appeared to be in a terrible mess, chopped about and distorted. I did not mention it, of course; to the ordinary eyesight his face looked perfectly normal, just as it always was. I left him then and went about my work, and he with his. A couple of days later I was on the phone to one of the parochial councillors, and he asked me if I had heard about their tragedy. I said I had not. He explained that the

verger had met with an accident. He had been working on a portable sawbench when the blade broke and flew up into his face. His face and head were badly cut, and he died on the way to hospital. Some weeks later when I visited that churchyard again, the verger's grave-stone was already in place – in the exact spot where he had been standing.

This sort of experience, when the inner feelings are open to the conscious awareness, goes a long way towards explaining how the dreaming process works, in particular this wholly unpredictable phenomenon of dreaming about future events. It may be that if, and only if, you are not able to become aware of some event while you are awake, it may be shown to you by way of dreams – if it is given to you to know about it.

A SENSE OF HUMOUR

Don't think that all dreams of the future relate to deadly serious matters or grim warnings. Some are light-hearted; a few are very obviously meant purely as 'a bit of fun'. What else can we make of the following example dream?

€ In the dream I was with an unknown man who seemed to be giving a lecture. We were walking through the house and he was standing just behind my shoulder, talking authoritatively about the project or experiment he was carrying out. I opened a door and we walked through into a room. There was a wide window-sill, on which was lying a man's head. Then I saw a table with a body lying on it, covered with a sheet. The lecturer said, rather pompously: 'In this experiment I set out to discover whether the head controls the body, or the body controls the head, and to this end I separated the head from the body. I have now discovered that the body cannot do without the head, and the head cannot do without the body, so I shall now put the head back on again'.

That was the end of the dream. The head had been lying on its side so that I saw it in profile, and it was very distinctive, like a caricature. It is still very vivid in my memory. Two days after the dream I opened the morning paper and there was a political cartoon – the sort where the characters have been given huge heads and tiny bodies – and there was the precise profile of the head and face in my dream, exact in every detail. It was a caricature of a well-known party leader!

115

DREAMS OF OTHER LIVES

I HAVE SPREAD MY DREAMS UNDER YOUR FEET;
TREAD SOFTLY, BECAUSE YOU TREAD ON MY DREAMS.

W.B. Yeats

*Y*OU may have discovered, as I and many others certainly have from personal experience, that it is possible some times to dream someone else's dream – quite unexpectedly; to experience *their* hopes and fears at first hand, in your own dream. It happens quite often when someone who is known to you personally, possibly somebody you care deeply about, chances for some reason to have occupied your immediate attention. For example, you may have been thinking a lot about a friend or relation, or they may have come to stay with you for a few days. Then one night you find to your surprise that you have inadvertently experienced something totally unique and personal to that individual: an intuitive dream, perhaps; a sort of thought-transference dream.

I dreamed I was driving my old car with a couple of friends, and we turned into the driveway of the local youth club, parked, and went inside. While we were there some lads who always cause trouble came in. They were a gang who threw their weight about a lot and were quite dangerous. Some people slipped out quietly when they came in, to avoid trouble. My friend was playing (or playing about) on the old piano that was there, and hadn't seen them arrive, so I stayed to keep him company, though I really wanted to get out. The gang leader came up to me and I tried to be casual and polite. He stood deliberately on my toe while I was talking, and it was very painful. I made some feeble joke about him having sharp shoes, or heavy feet, or something like that. Soon afterwards we managed to get out and left them to it.

It was not until a few days later that I realized this had been a true dream, not about me, but about a boy whom I knew and rather fancied. Perhaps I had been thinking or feeling emotionally about him that night. I found out that all the events in the dream had actually happened to him. I had not known that youth club even existed before, but a short time later I happened to pass the actual place – the driveway, the signboard and everything was exactly as I remembered it in the dream. I never made it with that boy, though, and I never even see him nowadays!

Nobody would suggest that this type of veridical, intuitive dream implies that the dreamer has actually *become* the other person. There is no question of experiencing 'reincarnation'; it is far more straightforward than that. For whatever reason, someone else's personal awareness, by way, probably, of their own unconscious sleeping self, has somehow impinged upon the blank sheet of your own awareness. You will have found out something about them that you could not otherwise possibly have known. It has happened to me several times over the years: you arrive at an understanding that was not there before and has not been arrived at through your own experience, or your own power of reasoning.

Quite often, dreams of this sort are best not recorded. They would in any case be meaningless without intimate knowledge of the person concerned. They may involve wholly confidential matters which, through the dreaming process, have been divulged to you alone.

SHARING THE EXPERIENCE

Even if you have not yourself dreamed of someone else's experiences, you might accept that this kind of confidential dream-sharing does sometimes happen. You may then wish to go a step further, and concede that such a dream might equally happen with regard to someone you *don't* know, someone whom you have *not* asked to stay for a few days, someone that you don't 'fancy', or feel emotionally about; someone perhaps from far away; someone even who may have lived many years before you were born. Well, of course, these dreams happen quite frequently too. You may not know the characters concerned, but does it make that much difference? Physical closeness may not be involved when dreaming of a complete stranger, but the dream will be no less 'solid' in its base, no less material. Time and space, involving the past, the present, the far away, the close at hand, are still concepts of materiality.

In a non-material world, which is the world we experience through our inner feelings in dreams, there seems to be no reason why time and space should be barriers to our shared experiences. The factors that cause you to dream of your friend's experiences seem likely to be similarities in the quality of feeling – parallel emotions or empathy, rather than physical proximity. In the first type of dream, the fact that you are close to one another physically suggests that thoughts and feelings of sympathy already in your mind and taken into your own inner feelings have triggered the dream. In dreams of the second type, a *compatible set* of thoughts and feelings have by chance been thrust upon your field of awareness.

Do you believe in reincarnation?

There is a strong body of opinion in the Western world nowadays that favours the idea of reincarnation: of personal continuation of life after death, in another body. As Hindus put it in poetic terms:

> The mind that flits like a butterfly through the garden of desires,
> sipping here and there and caring not for the future, flies to life
> and death again in the never-ending cycle of nature. A caterpillar,
> coming to the end of its leaf, reaches across and gains another leaf.
> The soul, leaving one body behind, reaches across and gains
> another body.

We know about the mysterious zone of the collective unconscious that surrounds us all and yet, in a strange way, seems to be included within the mind of our own self. If all selves are indeed linked in this way – and I certainly think they are – only a very short leap of faith is needed to make the assumption that all worldly experiences are related too. We know, through remembering our dreams, that the particularly traumatic experience of one person can be recalled and re-experienced, in the awareness of a different person. Experience will show that the griefs of other people – and griefs, it seems, are more likely to be shared than joys – are waiting to be shared, at some unknown level of the dreaming state.

OTHER TIMES, OTHER PLACES

A typical 'reincarnation' dream will be of people who are wholly unknown to you – obviously 'real' people, not to be confused with the 'imaginary' archetypal characters summoned up by your own subconscious mind – and you will be, not the old familiar 'you', but a different 'you'. Such a dream seems invariably to be centred around the psychological traumas of these complete strangers; perhaps their feelings of grief, experiencing the events leading up to their death, or to the death of someone else closely involved. Such dreams may be long and substantial, and are always strikingly vivid, often seeming to refer to a particular very definite time and place, or some well-known period of history.

It is not surprising that the dreamer is convinced that *they were that person* in another life, and they may go to great lengths to verify times and places and incidents, taking them as proof positive of reincarnation. There will indeed be little doubt that the original incident, the subject of the dream, actually took place; but of course it did *not* happen to the dreamer personally. The identifying feature is extreme emotional trauma – the factor that somehow imprinted a lasting record of a set of experiences, in the form of a solidly real dream continuing indefinitely as a separate, independent entity. Could that psychic record become established on a permanent cycle, somewhere at the outer rim of the sphere of collective awareness? I think so. It could then be picked up by any sensitive dreamer who chanced to be on the same empathic wavelength. The following example is just such a dream:

€ I seemed to be about seventeen years of age. I and about four ladies were getting out of a horse-drawn coach. We were all expensively dressed. We were being hurried out of the coach by a man on horseback. He wore a uniform with red tunic and white buckskin breeches. He was very well known to us in the dream, and I remember thinking how strange to see him with such very muddy, dirty breeches; he was usually immaculately dressed. We were outside a small inn, which was on the corner where two roads met. The horseman said: 'I am sorry to disturb you ladies. You will be all right, but we must have the horses.' The coach had been drawn by two horses, and another man had already taken them out of the shafts. Riding his own horse he cantered away, leading the two coach horses. Inside the inn we all gathered round a large table. An elderly couple (apparently the innkeeper and his wife) stood at one end of it. After a few moments we heard a tremendous clatter of horses, and we could see a great many men, who looked in through the window. We could see that they were Cromwell's troops. The innkeeper seemed very nervous. He grabbed his gun, which was in the corner near him, and fired blindly. I don't think he took aim. I heard a loud bang and felt myself falling, and realized I had been shot. There was some shouted conversation between the innkeeper and his wife. She was saying something like 'Oh, the poor thing!' and he was saying something like 'Well, they'll think we've been harbouring them!' That was the end of the dream.

This is not a dream that can be analysed, because it appears to carry no personal message for the dreamer; it is simply a record of the dramatic events leading up to a young girl's death, apparently some three and a half centuries earlier. The dreamer was positive that there had been no trigger events recently in her own life that might have aroused her creative imagination. She had not been reading about the English Civil War, or thinking about it in any way. This dream involved the apparent death of the dreaming personality, but it was the same dreamer, some years later when in her nineties, who had this equally vivid dream involving the death of another person:

I and another woman (I don't think I knew her) and a boy of about twelve were in an empty house, just looking around it. We had come up two flights of stairs, and we remarked what lovely big rooms they were. I said to the boy: 'There should be a lovely view of . . .' (I can't remember where I said), but when we looked through the window it was entirely different from what I had expected: just houses and fields. I walked back to the centre of the room. The boy suddenly opened the window and clambered on to the sill. I called to him to get down at once, but he just laughed and dangled his legs outside. He obviously thought it great fun to frighten me and the other woman. He got very excited and started rolling himself about on the sill. Suddenly he lost his balance and was gone. We both rushed to the window and looked out, and saw the boy lying in a sort of huddled heap, his legs on the paving and his head and shoulders practically under a hedge. I can't describe the horror and anguish I felt at seeing that small body lying there. I can still see his face, so round, happy and laughing, with fair wavy hair, with every promise of growing to be a handsome man. I remember he wore a shirt with blue and white squares. I felt guilty at having attracted his attention to the window in the first place.

We tried to analyse this dream, but again it yielded nothing, except the dreamer's own impression of a possible warning not to do or say something (however honestly meant) which, if followed, could lead to disastrous consequences. This is because she felt that, had she not mentioned the view, the boy would not have had the idea of climbing out on to the sill. The warning may well have been apt. Personally, however, I think this was purely 'another person's dream', a chance receiving on the communal wavelength, an empathic link across time and space, which contained no message, and no psychological significance, apart from itself.

There is little evidence in the dream that could point to a date; it did not seem to refer specifically to any particular time in the past, and, as the dreamer herself thought later, it could well have been contemporaneous in setting. The window, so the dreamer remembers, was of the sash rather than the casement type, and sash windows came into widespread popular use from the late seventeenth century. They were the commonest kind of window during the eighteenth century, but they are also, of course, still to be seen in many older houses today.

REMEMBERED NON-SELF DREAMS OF CHILDHOOD

Access to lost memories of childhood, long ago relegated to the personal unconscious, may come flooding back through dreams, and these are often too painful to relate. Within the family, all kinds of experiences may be shared within the often barely remembered dreaming process, particularly perhaps between parent and child, and probably far more commonly than we realize. As so much dreaming activity is in any case unconscious, we can guess that possibly 90 per cent of shared dreams will remain subliminal too, and fail to reach the waking mind. Of such dreams as do come to awareness, the waking experience of one member of the family may become the dream of another; you may find yourself dreaming your child's, your parent's, your brother's or your sister's dream. It is certainly not unusual for children to dream about their parents' problems or emotional disturbances, sometimes in realistic terms, seeing events from their parents' point of view, as if through their own eyes; sometimes in the imagery of disguise. The following was dreamed by a ten-year-old boy, accurately recalling something his father had experienced when he was the same age, some forty years earlier:

121

> ℂ It was during the First World War, when three or four soldiers were billeted on us. We were looking through a window into the garden. A very old, sick cat was walking slowly across the green lawn. It had been arranged that one of the soldiers should shoot the cat, to 'put it out of its misery', and he had his gun ready. He took aim and shot the cat dead, and I said: 'Got him!'

This was confirmed as a perfectly true account when the father happened to mention it some years later. The boy's story of his dream was not believed, naturally enough, his parents assuming he must have been told about the incident at some time. He on his part was adamant that he had not been told, and that it was a genuine dream experience.

Adults' memories of their own childhood dreams certainly are liable to have become confused with waking thoughts and imagination, but many seem too vivid and persistent to be other than genuine early dream experiences. This is an example of one such remembered dream from long ago, not a parent–child affair this time, but a 'reincarnation' memory:

> ℂ I was a Celtic man wearing a rough, hairy garment of some sort, and standing at the edge of the sea on a rocky shore. There was a Roman boat in difficulties some way out, and one of the young men was struggling to reach the shore. I don't think he was wearing the leather body armour that was a normal part of their uniform, though he had a scarlet tunic. Standing in the water, I thrust my spear into his midriff, and as he floundered dying in the waves he looked at me as though to say, 'Why? Why did you do that?' And I wondered too. I didn't know why.

BRIDGING THE BROAD GAP

The dreamer in the last example was in fact of Celtic descent. But very often 'reincarnation' dreams will cross racial boundaries. It is this sort of case that may cause the curious dreamworker to wonder if there has been a sexual link, a blending of inherited contents, to somehow bridge the gap and combine two distinct sets of ancestral experience. It is not difficult to imagine that two distinct individuals, two selves visualized as separate and independent mandalas, may become physically superimposed, so to speak, during normal male–female sexual relationships. Their unconscious contents at least may combine, or become able to be shared, whether the union is purely emotional or physical as well. The feelings certainly have to play a part: ancestral backgrounds may become merged on the level of the inner feelings, the source of dream expression.

€ In this dream I was on a lion hunt. I think it was an old rogue lion that had taken to killing cattle, and possibly people too. We knew it was lying up among some bush-covered rocks at the foot of a rocky hill, and about twelve of us with spears had the spot more or less surrounded. It was very hot. I could feel the sand hot between my toes. The other men were spread out in a semi-circle, advancing slowly without making a sound. Their bodies were shining with sweat. I knew them all, friends and neighbours. The rocks were quite vivid, shades of yellow, brown and grey. I looked back at my companions, all with their spears ready. I was among the rocks, and I realized that I was too far forward from the others, rather isolated and in danger, so I waited for them to draw level. Suddenly I saw the lion. He had a black mane, his rump was against the rock, and his head was raised in anger. I moved back and made the mistake of turning away for a moment. Then the others all shouted a warning together. I whirled round and tried to raise my spear, but it was too late, the lion was on me. I felt his crushing weight, his mane was smothering me and I smelled his choking smell. His claws fastened into my back, and his jaws clamped on my neck and the base of my skull.

It was not until long after I was awake and recalling the dream that I realized that I and all the others in the dream were tribal Africans. Although their faces were so familiar in the dream (and I remember some of those faces still), they were complete strangers to my waking self. I am an Englishman, and I dreamed the dream in England, though I did spend several years in the African bush, so in some ways I have been an 'honorary African'. I have since heard that black-maned lions, once common, have not been seen in the wild for several decades.

The dream was without doubt a re-run of somebody's last moments on earth. The faces of the other hunters were as real to the dreamer, within the dream experience, as those of the members of his family and his friends in real life. Once again, there is no real way that the dream could be interpreted, personally and specifically, in terms of day-to-day experience; and yet the dream itself was wholly personal and wholly specific – exact in detail and content. Retrospectively, the dreamer considers that the style of tribal dress would have placed the hunters no later than the decade before he was born – and he was born not in Africa, but in England. What then was the invisible link, and was the dreamer to consider it an actual case of reincarnation, or the sensitive sharing of a dreadful experience?

DO YOU STILL BELIEVE IN REINCARNATION?

In Chapter 5 we explored the technique of re-entering your dream, re-experiencing it, and extending or completing it, in order to understand it better. The strange experience of dreaming about other people's lives has encouraged the now well-known technique of hypnotic regression, which enables a dreamer apparently to return in time to the substance of a 'reincarnation' dream, to relive it and experience more

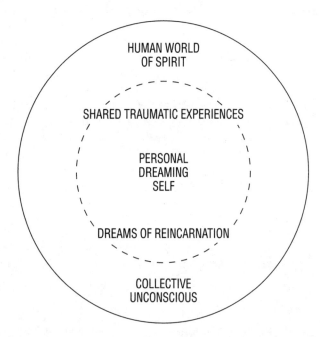

The 'personal' meets the 'impersonal'. To experience another's traumatic life-incident in your own dream is often taken as evidence of reincarnation. But the matter is put into perspective when you know that the other 'self', whom you experience in your dream, is still living.

of it, in greater detail. When positive results are obtained they do much to reinforce the basic belief, though a cynical bystander might remark that there is little practical difference, in principle or results, between the two techniques.

The diagram suggests a new way of looking at dreams of other lives. The personal self – yours, mine, theirs – sits in the centre of its own mandala, surrounded by two complementary and impersonal extremes: the collective unconscious, and the human world of spirit. Experience will show us, sooner or later, that close to the world of spirit, though there are dreams of shared trauma, they are not dreams of reincarnation.

'Empathy' means the ability to enter into another's experience. 'Compassion' means 'suffering with', and empathy and compassion provide the key to what such dreams are about. Empathy works when the dreamer is sensitive and open enough to receive the dream itself. Compassion is the result of the personal, individual passions becoming united – that is, when everything that can be felt about another person or their situation is able to be felt at the same time, when 'all things work together for good'. Empathy is necessary to experience something of the collective unconscious; true compassion belongs to the world of spirit, and it is always conscious.

My own conclusion, therefore, has to be that these apparently different types of dream – dreams of reincarnation, and dreams of shared disturbing experiences – are the same, of the same stuff. The only difference lies in the understanding of them, in the passions and perceptions of the dreamer. The sharing of trauma at this deep level is a personal and not a second-hand experience. In the dream itself there is no difference between 'reincarnation' and 'not reincarnation'. All are unique, yet all are united.

DREAMS OF DESTINY

DEEP INTO THAT DARKNESS PEERING,
LONG I STOOD THERE WONDERING, FEARING,
DOUBTING, DREAMING DREAMS NO MORTAL
EVER DARED TO DREAM BEFORE.

Edgar Allan Poe

URING the course of this book I have tried to put forward the concept of the inner feelings, the emotional contents of the unconscious mind, as that part of the self that seems to be working towards emotional wholeness. This subtle centre of being I see as the source of personal dream imagery and, as the go-between creating a balance between conscious and unconscious, spiritual and material, the selector of collective images and the collator of spiritual dreams. Soul-awakening means that these inner feelings can come to awareness as a non-egoistic self, quite independently of our normal ego, our everyday decision-making centre. If and when this happens to you, sleeping or awake, you will know that you have reached a major turning-point in your life.

It may have become fashionable to think of 'soul' as a theoretical idea connected with religious experience, or with a sense of cultural background, or with some special way of thinking, or emotional sensitivity, or some sort of inner power. The truth is, soul may include all those things, but it is not limited by anything like that. Soul represents the movement towards wholeness, and to this extent is to be identified with the experience of dreaming. It is aware not only of all aspects of ourselves, but it can see into others as well. Soul is familiar with both extremes: the dark contents of the subconscious, and the human world of spirit. If it happens that the inner feelings come to the surface of awareness, the source of personal dream imagery will automatically become available to the understanding too. That is when we are likely to experience 'dream imagery' while fully conscious and going about our daily business; we may experience intuitive 'waking dreams', such as the one described in Chapter 7.

Soul-awakening is not something you can do for yourself, and neither can anyone else do it for you: it may happen by itself if you are willing to accept it. You may discover the secret of it by yourself, but it might be more useful to inquire from the international organization known as Subud, or *Susila Budhi Dharma*, which exists for this purpose. Your primary concern will then be DESTINY.

SOUL-CHILDREN

Do you dream of your children? Even if you have no children in fact, do you still dream of them? These dream-children could be symbolizing separate aspects of your own soul: the children of your passions. When this soul family comes together, the personal self will have reached completion. The whole self has often been symbolized as a flower: in the West usually as a blue flower; in the East as a golden one. The complete 'human flower' with five petals represents your 'human family' – you are the whole flower, and the petals are your children. This type of flower, of course, is a form of mandala, another instinctively expressed picture of the self. If you superimpose this personal flower mandala on the world mandala, as overleaf, you will see that once again the correspondence is clear – the microcosm of the self relates to the macrocosm of the world.

Remember that these dream-children represent the different passions, different aspects of your own self. As a rule when you dream of them you will notice a difference between their individual complexions or hair colour – but naturally, as they are your own children, the details will depend largely upon your own racial type. The reason for this personal variation is to be found in the collective root of the dream: on the scale of the world dream they represent the whole of humankind, all the different racial types, and their colours reflect the fact that they are one human family: black, red, yellow, white, coming together as brown – a mixture of all the other colours. This is the symbology of the soul, the symbolic nature of the separate human passions which can unite to create compassion in the individual: the whole of the human race in the background of every single person. Our dreams will bring us to the discovery that we are all one family: we are all brothers and sisters 'under the skin', and we are all mothers

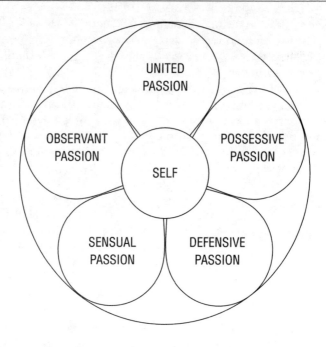

The flower mandala of the self. The five petals – the separate passions or parts of the personal soul – can feature in your dreams as children with differing characteristics.

or fathers of the human race – this is the symbolism of 'soul-children'. Don't let this piece of knowledge go to your head - it can open the door to a new way of thinking!

The 'passion of possession' often appears as the eldest child – usually of dark complexion, the most efficient and hard-working of the family, the practical child who can get things done. The 'passion of defence' is the next child by age, usually with a reddish complexion. This is the dream offspring who will watch out for your welfare, warning of any outsiders who may pose some sort of threat. The next child by age represents the 'passion of sensuality', usually with a sallow complexion, or fair with yellow hair. In your dreams this is a rather clever child who usually comes up with the answers, and who knows right from wrong. The next child in your personal family represents the 'passion of observation', and is usually seen as fair-complexioned, a child who always notices tiny details and, though so young, seems to understand human relationships very well.

There may even be a fifth child in this inner family – as a rule a brown-skinned baby, a very loving and beautiful child who represents all the rest of your family when it is at one in harmony. This child can only appear when the others are totally united, so they will probably not be seen all together. The others will perhaps not realize that this baby is their brother or sister too, because he or she represents their own potential. To dream of your own soul-family, as in the following example, is to take an inner look at your own self.

> In my dream I called at a farm to collect a young child whom they had been been looking after for me. I picked him up and got in the car ready to start off. I remember that he was fair-skinned, with blond hair. A younger child came out of the building with a toy car, smiling at me, and I was worried in case he strayed too far away, and told him: 'Go on back, your daddy's waiting!' The child turned back then. There was another person standing watching in the near distance. My child said: 'Oh, is that his daddy? He's a *lovely* baby!' I looked round then expecting to see my other older children, and saw them walking along the lane some distance away, two young men together. I thought there should be another one somewhere; then I saw him too, wearing a floppy hat and driving a herd of cows.

It is quite a common experience to dream of the self in this multiple way, for all the characters in this dream are parts of the dreamer's own self. The sensual passion is the part of the self most closely in tune with the world of animal nature, and this is the son who appeared in the dream attending to a herd of cows. The observant passion – the little boy collected by the dreamer – did not know that the baby with the toy car – the potential but undeveloped means of a new life's journey – was actually his own baby brother, or that he represented the family of passions united, the sum total of themselves. That union had not yet come about for the dreamer, but it was seen in the dream as a possibility for the future, when the baby is old enough to venture out on his own. When your personal passions really come together, they create compassion, or love, and only then will your mandala be complete.

YOUR DREAMS AS A CHILD

If you think about your own dream-family of children, you might see that it resembles yourself at different ages. As a newborn infant, too young to remember dreams but still, to all intents and purposes, actually living in 'dreamland', you were that sweet and loving brown-skinned baby, not yet fragmented into separate passions. As a toddler you were that fair-haired child, watching how grown-ups and older children do things, starting to learn about the world, and your dreams at that age will have reflected this stage of development. Then you were that golden, animal-loving kid, learning how to get on with other children and find your true place in the world, and these things featured in your dreams at that time. As a rather older child you were that ruddy-complex-ioned youth apt to boss people around a little, fierce in competitive sports and other pursuits, and this was the kind of action you dreamed about. Later still as a teenager, you were that dark and serious young person who was already adept at so many things, who had probably already plotted out your future career. Your dreams will have reflected your own familiarity with *things*, with tools and sports equipment, cars, bicycles, motorcycles, clothes, and your own status in society.

As an adult, if you meet with the possibility of rediscovering your own soul-life, you will begin to reverse this process, to re-experience these stages of soul development. Symbolically, you will be growing younger, and this is when you are likely to dream of your own family of the self. If you refer back to the world mandala, you may see all this as a descent from birth through the human stage, the animal stage and the plant stage, finally reaching the material stage. The long climb back through these levels of soul-life is expressed, or symbolized, in various ways by the different religions and philosophical systems – a slow climb back to the pure condition where you will have become 'again like a little child'. Many dreams reflect your own inner understanding of this jour-ney, and it can be expressed in numerous different ways, depending on your own experiences and expectations in life. This is another example:

In the dream I was about ten or twelve years old, and was sitting on a hearth-rug with two other little girls about the same age, and I was excitedly telling them what I had just seen. There were some new people moving into a house just near us, and I was standing outside watching the furniture van being unloaded. As the men were getting a sort of cupboard out, one of them slipped, and the cupboard banged on the side of the van, knocking a piece of wood off – only a thin piece, but, can you believe it – underneath this knocked-off layer I could see that it wasn't wood, but flesh, like beef in a butcher's shop, and while I watched, it started to bleed. This is what I told the girls. We were all rather excited, and wondered if perhaps the new people were witches who had turned people into furniture!

I woke up at dawn feeling very fresh and exhilarated, as if I had just bounced down like a balloon. I actually felt the bounce as I woke up. Remembering the dream afterwards, the feeling of happiness and exhilaration lasted for a long time after waking up, during the day. Of the two other little girls in the dream, one had been fair with yellowish curly hair. The other was more plain and dark or mousey. They wore pinafores with white frilly tops (like I used to wear as a child). The hearth-rug we were sitting on was darkish brown with no particular design.

This dream carries the message that the soul-child (the dreamer) is climbing back towards the point of childhood, towards the pristine human state, has attained the level of the animal world, the spiritual status of a ten year-old, and is approaching the exalted human state. The weird symbol of furniture that has flesh and can bleed seems to express the transition from the 'animal', through the 'plant', to the 'material' level of the soul. It suggests that a material dream-object, a cupboard fashioned out of wood – or plant material – still mysteriously contains the principle of animal life. Children can be 'little devils', but their spiritual level is quite exalted compared with the solidly material world of the adult. Childhood levels of being may be left far behind, but they are never really lost. Potentially, they can always be regained.

JOURNEY TO A DARK VALLEY

There is no getting away from the world dream, expressed by the world mandala, because it forms the background, setting the scene for dreams of the soul life. Our dreams express what is happening inside us: whether they seem to be purely about sex, or everyday relationships, or anxious situations, they are inner portraits. We can see now that *all* dreams are really 'soul dreams'. Some dreams are frightening indeed, others reassuring. Perhaps the difference depends on our own inner orientation – whether this is aimed towards strengthening our solidity, allowing the needs of materiality to dictate our actions, or in the opposite direction, towards a more childlike simplicity. Religions of the world are full of images expressing the ease with which people can go 'the wrong way'. There seems to be a great deal of confusion about. But we seldom want to take someone else's word for anything so important, and it is good if we can find out for ourselves the best course and attitude to take. Dreams can help: I believe that is their ultimate purpose. The following example seems to symbolize the unfortunate results that may follow an extreme course of action:

   [ℇ] I was sorry to hear about a former colleague of mine who had recently committed suicide – I have no idea what drove him to it. I know this dream was about him, though I did not actually see him in the dream, but in it I had the notion that I ought to go and visit him, and set out to do so. I found myself walking in some sort of deep valley which was filled with heavy fog. It seemed a barren place, strewn with rocks. I could see the ruins of one or two stone buildings through the fog, and it seemed to me that I was getting close to where I wanted to go. But it was all very puzzling, and then I became strongly aware that there were packs of fierce dogs running wild in that valley, and felt very scared, so I decided to come back up out of the fog and return to safety. That is when I woke up.

WALKING INTO THE LIGHT

By our very nature as adult human beings, most of us are psychically centred within or very close to the region of materiality – materiality is the principle, like it or not, that rules our lives. Nobody really knows what conditions are like in the upper half of the world mandala – in the world of spirit. It is out of our ken. Many people, certainly, have reported 'out-of-body' experiences, 'near-death' experiences, 'after-life' experiences – experiences which merge into dreams – and their accounts range from a dark and terrible place on the one hand, to a light and delightful place on the other. From what I have learned so far about dreams, *it seems to me* that both these extremes are to be found at the place where we live, for they already exist within our own selves – within this world zone of materiality. The experience of 'walking into the light' is certainly very close indeed to a place of darkness, as this (rather typical) example dream, following a death in the family, shows:

   [ℇ] I dreamed I was walking with my husband along a country road when it suddenly grew dark, and then became pitch black. I could no longer see him, and we got separated. I just kept calling and feeling about, but to no avail, so I just kept trudging on and on through the dark. After a very long time I saw a faint glimmer of light, which appeared to come from two narrow windows on either side of a door. It seemed to be a small church or chapel. I put my hand on the door and it opened a little, so I went in, thinking there might be someone in there who could help me. It was a bit lighter inside. As soon as I

132

went in I was grabbed by a lot of goblin-like creatures (in the dream I thought of them as 'goblins') who held my arms and pushed me at speed down the nave, while many more of them jumped over the pews on either side. They kept making a frightening jabbering noise. They rushed me at great speed as far as the altar, then back up the nave just as fast. On reaching the door again they let me go, and I escaped as quickly as possible.

Then, standing outside in the pitch dark, I suddenly saw another door open, as though across the road, showing a brilliant light. Three or four people were trooping slowly in. I dashed across the road to ask them where I was, but then as I reached the door I saw my husband standing a few feet inside, so I ran in. I was so excited, I grabbed his arm and asked him: 'What are you doing here?' He said: 'I was waiting for you.' I said: 'But how did you know I'd be coming here? I was lost; I might never have found you.' He just said calmly: 'Oh, I knew you'd come.' We wandered off arm in arm, and I said: 'This is such a beautiful place, flowers everywhere, and everyone so happy.' My husband said, 'It's called the "Elysian Fields".' We walked on very happily. Then I became aware that I was dreaming, and fell into a deep dreamless sleep.

There are so many vivid accounts of dreams, or out-of-body experiences, involving 'walking into the light' that we can be sure they are not all mere fantasy. But then, fully formulated dreams are *not* fantasy. Walking into brightly lit rooms full of welcoming people; strolling through fields of beautiful flowers; meeting deceased relatives in an aura of love: all these have been described as experiences of 'heaven'. But remember the principle of moving with the flow of the world dream, rather than against it. These wonderful images, these regions of light, can be found symbolized within the world mandala by the material segment as it extends above the horizon. It is, in effect, the state of materiality bathed in an archangelic light. Our normal everyday psychic 'centre of gravity' is already there, within the region. When a dream door swings open, it is but a short step for us to enter that light.

Such a vision, if it can be described in physical terms, may be a glimpse of 'paradise', but it cannot truly be called an out-of-body experience of 'heaven'. Words tend to lose their power when we try to make the distinction, because we have no experience of those realms symbolized by the uppermost segments of the world mandala. 'Heaven' has no basis for description within our familiar terms of reference; no images that our earthly minds can grasp or hold. The

'Elysian Fields' that you enter, therefore, should not be confused with a truly spiritual experience.

The flow of evolution leads from the barren rock of materiality, through the lower life forms, plants and animals, to and beyond the human creation, to complete the world cycle within unknown realms. We have seen how people develop from birth, growing away from a childish state towards an adult mastery of materiality. And when that has been achieved to the best of our ability, our dreams hint at the necessity for a return to source; a need to submit to that gentle current. Our dreams may portray this journey as a long, lonely path that leads – who knows where? Yet when the full sequence of our dreams is made clear to us, we can see that this way, though strewn with difficulties, is the one we *ought* to be following.

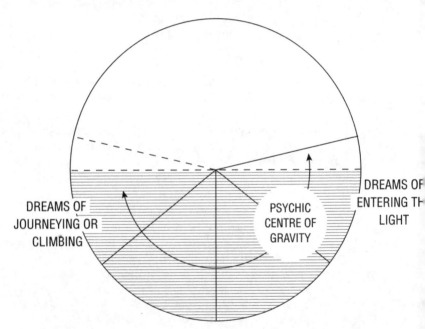

In dreams involving death – either your own or that of somebody else – you may experience entering a pleasant place full of light. This also happens quite often during 'near-death' experiences. Our study of the world dream suggests that the light symbolizes a 'paradise' within the confines of materiality. Dreams which feature a long and difficult journey or steep climb, however, symbolize an inner journey towards a more exalted, saintly condition.

You cannot do it yourself

Forget, once and for all, the popular notion of 'spiritual power'. There is no such thing, as far as we mortals are concerned. In the words of the psalm, 'Power belongeth unto God.' Supernatural power on earth belongs to the realm of the occult, and occult practices run against the grain of spiritual experience. If you personally have had anything to do with the occult, or power on a supernatural plane – by trying to make things happen with or within the subtle, non-physical side of yourself – you may find a stern warning arriving in the form of a dream. This was the experience of a thirty-five-year-old man who had met with the possibility of soul-awakening, of commencing the long journey 'back to base', and he was determined to try to follow it. But in the past he had been interested in the occult, and now made the mistake of deliberately trying to accelerate the purifying process.

As we all know by now, the natural cycle of dreams works towards stirring and bringing out the dark, unseen contents of the subconscious into the open, into awareness, gradually bringing symbolic light to the whole self rather than merely the upper half. People who practise the occult sometimes claim to be able to control this balancing-out process themselves with their own will, by exorcizing, or conjuring up and expelling, the dark images that have taken up residence in the recesses of our own unconscious minds – our own personal demons; our own shadow.

> ℂ I thought I had got rid of the unwanted contents of my own sub-conscious mind, and went to sleep feeling quite light and psychologically free. But I dreamed I heard the sound of someone casting out a devil, and this devil was walking around and visiting all the people I knew, trying to get accepted into them, but without success. Personally in the dream I felt secure against it. Then in my dream the bedroom door was pushed open and our family pet walked in – a very large, affectionate and overweight boxer dog – and came up to the bed and nuzzled me. I stroked and petted the dog and felt glad it was there. But then my hand felt that the dog's hairs had turned into coarse bristles and it was not really a dog at all; I was caressing a demonic sort of dog-creature that reared its head and gave me a terrifying stare. As I woke up it slowly faded from view. It seemed to be still there and still fading away as I was fully awake in the dawn light, and my hair was standing on end. I felt bitterly cold, and I have never felt so frightened in my life. I had just welcomed back my own pet demon!

GUILT - OR DOUBLE MEANINGS

In my own experience, if you are a receptive sort of person and your dreams are progressing well, it may seem to you that you have been called upon to act as a 'confessor' for someone known to you, who is about to die; to dream of their guilt by proxy. This is quite logical: it is not good to die with feelings of guilt, for it seems that such feelings can hamper your progress after death. They can impede your long walk or climb towards the pristine state of wholeness. Certainly dreams bear this out. Shortly before my own neighbour was killed in a road accident, I had the following very vivid dream:

> ☾ In this dream I was at a farm, and the farmer and farm workers had cleared out the bales and produce from a large stone-built barn. The remaining straw and chaff was fairly full of rats, and the workers set fire to this litter and sealed all the doors and windows, to kill the rats. I could hear them frantically clawing at the doors, leaping and scuffling as they tried to escape. I thought it was extremely cruel, and felt very upset and guilty about it, but there was nothing I could do about it. The farmer saw my distress and tried to turn it into a joke, pretending that the rats were dancing inside. 'Don't you worry,' he said. 'They're having the time of their lives!' I thought this was even worse; to joke about it. They may have been 'only rats', but that is no reason to be unnecessarily cruel.

As I woke, half asleep still, I worried at first about the terrible guilt I felt for something that had absolutely nothing to do with any experience or act on my own part, and I exonerated myself from all blame. Nobody under those circumstances could really have influenced the outcome. As though I were speaking to someone else, I said: 'No, you are absolutely free of blame. You were not at fault. No guilt attaches to you.' And I suddenly felt free of that guilt which I seemed to have taken on, because of someone else's cruelty.

It then came to me, very powerfully, that it was my neighbour and not me who had experienced the reality of that dream, probably a boyhood experience, and shared those feelings with me. There is no doubt in my mind who the real owner of that dream was, and when I heard of his death a couple of days later I hoped that my 'forgiveness' of that undeserved feeling of guilt would help the future progress of that kind-hearted man. It seemed to have fallen to me to take that guilt, experience it, and then disown it and abolish it.

But wait! What about the double meaning? Look at it from another point of view. Suppose the barn represents the dreamer's (and in this case, my own) subconscious mind, and the tormented rats symbolize the unwanted traits and peccadillos, or the 'astral parasites' to which we may all be involuntary hosts. It is normal, if not inevitable, that a person will want to keep his or her own contents, to remain wholly attached, through intimate familiarity, to traits that others would see as undesirable faults. If those faults seem on the point of being cleaned out or neutralized, such a person will naturally feel upset and agitated. Subconscious contents become a real part of the whole person as he or she *is*, and it can be extremely painful to lose them. But whose barn was it, in this particular case – mine, or my neighbour's? Many dreamworkers would interpret the dream in this personal way, and dismiss my idea of 'confessing' someone else's unwanted characteristics as a mistake bordering on arrogance. But *I* say it is all part and parcel of sharing at a deeply human level. My awareness of the impending death of my neighbour may seem to militate against a personal interpretation, but both versions may be simultaneously correct.

You will probably already have observed that there are often at least two ways of understanding many dreams. Suppose, for instance, you dream that you need the toilet quickly, but can only find ones that don't work, or are too disgustingly dirty to use, or are too much in the public eye, or turn out to be incomplete, or unusable in some other way. This is quite a common dream. It may mean simply that you have a physical need to go urgently, and your own ego is arguing with your inner feelings, the one saying, 'I want to go now!' and the other saying, 'You can't, because you are still asleep in bed!' The physical explanation is simple enough. But certainly, if you don't actually need to wake up and go to the toilet at that time, there must be another explanation: the need for shedding impurities, psychically, spiritually. You have character defects, perhaps, which you know ought to be expelled, but you will find any excuse for hanging on to them a bit longer. As the first St Augustine wrote in his *Confessions*, 'Give me chastity . . . but do not give it yet.'

CLIMBING TOWARDS ETERNITY

Many people dislike speaking of the concept of 'purgatory', believing such ideas to be speculative and sectarian. But this is mainly a quarrel about terms, about words, rather than concepts. 'Purgatory', or purification, is simply a convenient name for the long-drawn-out process of turning out and discarding the psychic rubbish that has accumulated in our darker depths. If you make a mistake in your thinking, this can quite easily be corrected. As soon as you learn the truth about some matter, your previous erroneous opinion can be modified, or abandoned and forgotten. Similarly with emotional feeling; if you are attached to someone or something that proves unreliable, or unlovable, your feelings towards that person or thing will change. The change in this case will not be so quick and painless as a mere change of mind, but a change of heart will happen eventually. But the inner feelings which show themselves in dreams run much more deeply than our everyday hearts and minds, and are not to be reached by our normal conscious awareness.

Purgatory symbolically describes the process of turning our personal sphere, half darkness and half light, into all light, while the passions that normally motivate us during our lives are inoperative. It is like climbing out of our own dark pit. We have seen how every impression or influence we meet during our lives sinks into the unconscious part of our being, where at this hidden level unwanted contents accumulate until they affect the quality of the whole person – the potentially whole people that we are. Many vivid dreams have reflected this climbing-out process continuing after the death of a friend or loved one. The dream that follows is typical of the sort, and was recorded by a recently widowed mother of four grown-up sons.

I and my four boys were standing near a window, and about a yard away from it was a very, very deep chasm. The side of the chasm was almost perpendicular, and we could see that here and there people were struggling to climb up it. As we watched, I was amazed to see my husband just managing to climb out. In front of him now was a very, very steep hill, completely black, without grass or colour of any kind. We could see people climbing it until they disappeared into a thick white cloud. We were all very excited to see my husband, the boys' father, and we opened the window and called to him. I said the boys could push a ladder across the chasm, and he could crawl along it, and come in through the window, but he said: 'No, if I tried that I'd only fall down and have to climb all the way up again!' He didn't seem at all upset. In fact he looked quite exhilarated, as though enjoying himself, as he turned and started to climb up the steep black hill. We stood there watching until he disappeared from view into the thick white cloud. I woke up then.

138

It would be difficult to find a better example or a clearer dream-picture of the long final climb of the soul. Taken at its face value, it is very much a 'for your information' rather than a 'wishful thinking' dream. Wishful thinking would be far more likely to conjure up a vision of those sunlit fields or that bright welcoming room; a 'false heaven' within the material sphere. Our dream studies suggest that there is only one way to 'heaven' proper – a way that involves a long and lonely and, it seems, an exhilarating struggle. If you refer back to Chapter 3 you will find a sequel to this dream, which seems to be indicating to the dreamer that a climb such as this is not really a matter of choice.

In dreams our sense of 'self' loses its concrete edge. There seems no doubt that truly personal dreams represent some condition, some process that is happening inside ourselves, often at a very deep level. But what are we to think when the dream really seems to be indicating or illustrating something happening to another person? In terms of the inner self, it seems, we have *become* that other person, in an honorary capacity. The more inward, the more 'spiritual' the dream, the more will that non-self experience be shared until, carried to the ultimate degree, all people can be seen as one entity with mutual experiences.

Such a state of unity can be symbolized by the soul-children of your dreams – the various races of humankind – becoming united in one all-loving brown child; the whole world uniting in harmony. A remote possibility, to be sure; but this should be the spiritual goal for us all. To dream of another's troubles, discoveries and non-material progress, whether before or after the mysterious transition we call death, is to this extent a spiritual experience. To respect our dreams is to move in the right direction.

INDEX OF DREAM SYMBOLS AND IMAGES

GENERAL INDEX